HUMAN HORIZONS SERIES

LIVING WITH MENTAL ILLNESS

A Book for Relatives and Friends

ELIZABETH KUIPERS, BSc, MSc, PhD, FBPSS
PAUL BEBBINGTON, MA PhD, FRCP, FRCPsych

A CONDOR BOOK
SOUVENIR PRESS (E&A) LTD

The right of Elizabeth Kuipers and Paul Bebbington to be identified as authors of this work has been asserted by them in accordance with the Copyright, Designs and Patents Act 1988.

First published 1987 by Souvenir Press (Educational & Academic) Ltd, 43 Great Russell Street, London WC1B 3PA and simultaneously in Canada

Reprinted 1989, 1997, 2002
Third edition 2005

ISBN 0 285 637 41 X

Typeset by FiSH Books, London
Printed and bound in Great Britain by MPG Books, Bodmin, Cornwall

Contents

Preface to the Third Edition

It is now nearly twenty years since we first wrote this book. In that time there have been major changes in the National Health Service, not least in mental health services. The move towards community treatment has accelerated, and the important role of relatives in the care of people with severe mental illness has now been formally recognised in a series of government initiatives. This means that the attitudes of professionals towards carers have improved considerably, but not that services for them are uniformly better.

It was in this context that we revised the book in 1997, which now describes and takes account of these new developments. We have taken the opportunity of this reprinting to make further revisions and to remove sections that are out-dated. We hope that this third edition will still be of use.

Elizabeth Kuipers
Paul Bebbington
London, April 2005.

Foreword for the Second Edition

My father, Reggie Dingwall (1908–2003), who originally suggested writing this book and who sponsored the first edition, was no stranger to hard knocks, but he often managed to turn bad experiences into something positive. He spent his childhood in a vicarage in the south of England where he was misdiagnosed as having cancer. At the age of 8, he had to regularly travel to London, often on his own, for 'x-ray treatment'. He survived the treatment and went on to study anthropology at Oxford before going out to Africa to work for the Sudan Political Service for nearly 25 years. During the war he was, as he put it, 'invalided into the army' for a short spell while recovering from yellow fever. There he had time to do some stamp collecting, which he took up again after retirement to raise money out of 'waste paper' for the Sudanese Church. Over the years a team of helpers formed, many of whom found sorting stamps for a good cause very helpful in their own lives.

My parents married after the war. Their first child was born severely handicapped and died at the age of two. Shortly thereafter my mother had her first 'breakdown'. Reggie stood by her while she went through various forms of treatment and they had three other children. With the help of medication my mother managed to maintain a fairly normal life with several stays in hospital, but she often tried to stop taking her tablets, sometimes without telling him. At that time, mental illness was rarely discussed openly and my father had few people he could talk to about it apart from the professionals, who seldom had much time. But he and my mother were lucky to have had some supportive family and friends.

My mother died in a mountain accident in 1980 and a few months later my sister, who had also suffered from mental illness, committed suicide. During this difficult time of mourning my father impressed me greatly by, for example, spending time with people who were desperately keen to help him, even when he might have preferred to be with closer friends. He had time to reflect back on how he had tried to look after my mother and sister, and realised that it would have been easier if he had been better informed and if he had realised that so many other people caring for their 'sick' partners and relatives had similar worries. This was when my brother, father and I started to discuss the idea of a book to help the friends and relatives of people with mental illness.

Many people have told us over the years how this book by Elizabeth Kuipers and Paul Bebbington has helped them. This, in turn, has helped us to come to terms with some of the sadnesses of the past. If you are reading this now, then it may be because you are having to deal with a difficult and worrying situation. My hope is that you will find some of the answers to your questions from this book and glean some reassurance from it, and also that you will feel encouraged to talk to others about your problems and to look after yourself too. I wish you the best of luck in finding support and in caring for your sick friend or relative.

Silvia Dingwall, March 2005

Foreword to the First Edition

This book was written in memory of two members of our family who suffered from mental illness. Our experiences with them made us appreciate the need for something written specially for those confronted by mental illness in someone close to them. We put the idea to the Mental Health Foundation, who asked Dr. Kuipers and Dr. Bebbington to write this book. We hope that the result of their enthusiasm and hard work may encourage relatives and friends.

Above all, we hope that it will help them to realise that they are not alone, and that many are facing similar experiences.

Reggie, Brian and Silvia Dingwall

The Authors

Elizabeth Kuipers is Professor of Clinical Psychology at the Institute of Psychiatry and holds an Honorary post as a Consultant Clinical Psychologist in one of the Community Mental Health Teams of the South London and Maudsley NHS Trust. She trained in Psychology and Clinical Psychology at the Universities of Bristol and Birmingham respectively, and holds a Doctorate from London University. She has a particular interest in the problems of families who live with a person who has psychosis, and in psychological treatments for people with psychosis. She has published many articles in scientific journals and several other books.

Paul Bebbington is Professor of Social and Community Psychiatry at Royal Free and University College London where he is Head of the Department of Mental Health Sciences. He is also an Honorary Consultant Psychiatrist with the Camden & Islington Mental Health and Social Care NHS Trust, currently working with a prison mental health inreach team. He was trained in medicine at Cambridge University and St Bartholomew's Hospital in London, and in psychiatry at the Maudsley. He is particularly interested in the social aspects of depression and psychosis. He has written or edited a number of scientific books, and has published widely in scientific journals.

Introduction

This book is intended for the carers of people affected by severe mental ill health. Everybody knows of someone who has had a 'nervous breakdown', and for large numbers of us this means someone in the family. Even so, mental illness is more widespread than most people realise. Not everyone is affected in the same way, or to the same extent. In this book we have concentrated on the problems you may face if your relative suffers from the more severe mental disorders called psychoses: basically **schizophrenia**, **manic depressive illness** or **bipolar disorder**. These are among the most severe mental health conditions, but even so are much more common than most people think. It is estimated, for instance, that more than a quarter of a million people in this country suffer from either chronic or relapsing schizophrenia. This is like the population of a medium sized city, Derby for example. To put it another way: in Britain perhaps four people every day suffer a first attack of schizophrenia. Manic depressive illness is even more common. Where we work in inner London, it is reckoned that about 15% of local people will be treated by a psychiatrist for depression at some time in their lives, although most of them will suffer relatively mild forms of the disorder. Psychiatrists do, of course, deal with other disorders, but these are mostly less severe, or, like dementia, begin towards the end of life, and result in a different set of problems.

Living with someone always takes a certain amount of skill, and tensions arise from time to time in even the best-ordered relationships. Not everyone is equally good at this, but most people manage to keep their relationships going reasonably satisfactorily. We learn to do this from a young age, by watching others and by having our own, sometimes temporary, friendships. However, if you live with someone who develops a psychosis, whether schizophrenia or bipolar disorder, you are almost certain to be presented with problems that you have never met before, and that you may never even have heard about from anyone else. Some people in this situation are lucky, and hit on good ways to cope with it from early on. Others don't cope so well, and this may lead to further and increasing difficulties. They often then blame themselves for the way things have turned out. While this is understandable, it is not appropriate. If there were the equivalent of college courses in how to live with someone suffering from a severe mental illness, it would perhaps be a different matter, but there aren't. In fact, although things are improving, there is still not much guidance, so people try to adapt their previous experiences to deal with the new situation. Unfortunately, this new situation is so different from anything they have previously known that old and tried methods of coping may not work. It is because schizophrenia and bipolar disorder can lead to difficulties of a rather particular and persistent kind, both for people with severe mental health problems and for their carers, that we have written this book.

The policy of community care for people with mental illness is now around fifty years old. The driving force in the last century was that mentally ill people should no longer be kept for long periods in old and poorly maintained mental hospitals. Instead, facilities were to be developed in the community – day-hospitals, psychiatric wards in local general hospitals, day-centres, group homes, hostels and the like. However, it took time for these new facilities to be introduced. The result was that the hard work of caring for the mentally ill fell increasingly upon relatives or carers. Even now, the provision of community mental health services is not uniformly good throughout the country, and services may be seriously overstretched in many areas, particularly the inner cities, but also in some rural communities.

Although living at home has many potential benefits, psychiatrists and other health professionals are very concerned about the effects that severe mental illness has on the lives of sufferers and their carers. In our last preface, we were somewhat pessimistic about the way community care imposed additional burdens on carers, but we think services have improved appreciably over the last ten years. Nevertheless, we hope you will still gain support and help from this book.

While medication is important, the management of severe psychiatric problems has always required more than straightforward pill-pushing by doctors. People with severe mental ill health need to be offered services that they feel are appropriate. There is now considerable emphasis on patient choice and empowerment and collaborative relationships. Discussions between professionals and service users may concern ways in which they might adjust their lifestyle in order to keep well. This may involve organising work, leisure and educational activities, and types of supported housing like hostels or supported flats. It is also recognised that people do better if their care is the responsibility of a named person over a considerable period of time – the principle of 'continuity of care'.

Since the early 1990s, the basis of community care has been the 'Care Programme Approach' (CPA). This laid down guidelines for mental health teams which still apply. An important part of this approach is the involvement of service users and carers in planning for future care. The Government introduced a 'National Service Framework' in 1999, which not only emphasised the role of carers, but insisted that the mental health services should assess the needs of each carer on a yearly basis. This represents the final part of a radical change in the attitudes of mental health professionals towards carers.

There have been other very important changes over the last ten years. The research (almost all British) into psychological treatments for severe mental disorder has certainly led to a change of view. There is now more emphasis on the overlap between the psychological processes involved in even severe mental ill health, and the psychological processes of mentally healthy people. In other words, the symptoms of severe mental ilness represent an extreme combination of relatively common mental experiences and normal thought processes. Emphasising this may have the effect of making the illnesses more acceptable to the people who have them and to their carers, and perhaps eventually to the population at large.

If you live with someone who has psychosis, you will have many questions you would like answered. We have tried to think what these might be, and to answer them. The first chapter is mainly concerned with basic information about severe mental illness. The next deals with the difficulties you may have to face in living with someone who suffers from problems of this type. Following this, two chapters are devoted to various types of services and treatments. The fifth chapter covers the legal processes surrounding compulsory admission and treatment, and the safeguards that are

built into the 1983 Mental Health Act, and the legislation
introducing Community Supervision orders. The Mental Health Act
is due to be revised shortly, although there have been considerable
delays in doing this. The last chapter considers the feelings you
might have about your situation and how you might cope with them.
At the end of the book is a short list of useful web sites and an
index. We have decided to leave out the Chapter on benefits, as
these change quite quickly and it is now relatively easy to get advice
about these from other sources.

We hope that a quick glance will tell you whether the book will
help you. You are bound to have questions we have not covered, so
do not be afraid to ask the people treating and caring for your
relative for answers and advice. It is essential to realise that you
have an important part to play in your relative's recovery. Although
you may sometimes find things discouraging, helping your relative
can also be very rewarding, and it may be vital for them.

Severe mental illness is a field in which there are still many
uncertainties. You may still come across professionals with very
differing views on particular subjects, and some will put them
forward with total conviction! If you are not aware of this, it can be
especially confusing. Sadly, although things have improved
considerably in the nearly twenty years since the first edition of this
book, many professionals remain unclear about how best to deal
with the difficulties you may experience in living with someone
who has a severe mental health problem. In fact, you are an expert
in this field, in the sense that you have first hand experience, and
you may perhaps have already tried many of the suggestions that
might be made to you.

We have tried to avoid the appearance of being certain when we
aren't. After all, each person's situation is different. However, the
suggestions we make have been found useful by other people in
similar circumstances, and may work for you.

Finally, in the book we give examples from the situations and
experiences of clients and relatives we have known. We think
personal anecdotes add colour to what we have to say, and you may
be able to identify with some of the stories. However, in the
interests of confidentiality, we have disguised the identities of all
the people we write about.

1 Severe Mental Illness

Mental illness is a broad term that covers the problems that some people have in connection with the way they think, feel or behave. It includes several different conditions, and their effects can vary from states of relatively temporary distress to long-lasting problems. In this book we have chosen to focus on the more severe disorders.

It is sometimes difficult to distinguish mild states, for instance, of anxiety or depression, from ordinary experiences, and indeed the transition from what we think of as normal to the definitely abnormal is a gradual one. This is made more complicated because 'abnormal' can mean two different things: what is abnormal for a given person, and what would be abnormal for anyone. In general, we tend to think of mental states as abnormal when the person is clearly and persistently unable to function properly in society as a result. This is important because, once we recognise that someone is mentally unwell, we are quite rightly prepared to make allowances for them, at least to some extent, in a way we wouldn't if we thought they were merely misbehaving, or fooling about, or just being rather self indulgent. This distinction can be an issue even in the more severe psychiatric conditions that are the subject of this book.

For most of us, mental illness is a disturbing and frightening thing. This is partly because people who are mentally ill can behave in unpredictable, unfamiliar and sometimes embarrassing ways. It is particularly distressing when these changes happen to someone close to us. Worst of all, the mentally ill make us feel helpless – the normal ways of helping people do not seem to work. It is hurtful and confusing when we try to be sympathetic and supportive, and to offer constructive advice, only to find it ignored, rejected, or even seriously misinterpreted.

It has often been said that mental illnesses are illnesses like any other. This is not quite true though: for instance, we do respond to illnesses of the mind in a rather special way. When someone is physically ill, there is no problem about understanding their behaviour, because we see the reason for it: we might behave the same way in similar circumstances. However, it may be impossible to uncover the reasons why mentally ill people behave as they do. Sometimes, the reasons are based on beliefs that appear wrong-headed, or are obviously untrue. Individuals may also claim to have experiences which seem to be quite fantastic or absurd. This is upsetting, and it is not surprising that people shy away from the topic. They often use euphemisms like suffering from nerves or nervous breakdown to describe mental conditions.

For these reasons, mental illness is still associated with many myths and misunderstandings. Those who have had mental health problems may feel, often with justification, that they are shunned and stigmatised by society. When we first wrote this book we felt that these attitudes were beginning to change. However, over the last twenty years progress has not been smooth. Both in the 1990s and more recently, tragedies in which members of the public were killed by people with severe mental disorders were greeted by the most appalling headlines in tabloid newspapers. Attempts by clinicians and carers alike to provide more information and encourage more open attitudes faced an uphill battle in the face of media exploitation like this. However, when the boxer Frank Bruno recently developed a mental illness, the Sun newspaper was forced to back-track very rapidly from a callous headline announcing the fact. It quickly set up an appeal for a mental health charity, and was clearly embarrassed by the bad publicity and the angry response of its readers. Thus a blow may have been struck against the purveyors of stigma, aided not least by the dignified response of Mr Bruno when he recovered. Likewise, an American hospital soap opera, based in New York but attempting to copy the popular ER, was pulled off the air after its first episode portrayed a sensationalised storyline about violence in the context of mental illness. So the angels sometimes win.

Psychiatrists and psychologists cannot rely on any simple investigation, like a blood test, for finding out if someone has a particular mental health problem, although there is now good evidence that the more severe forms may be associated with subtle changes in brain chemistry. This being so, they can only recognise particular sorts of mental ill health from the way people behave and the things they say. This business of recognising which problem someone has is called 'diagnosis'. Doctors treating physical illnesses always feel it is important because, in theory at any rate, it narrows down the possibilities – the course the illness will take, the proper treatment to give, the likely response to it, and so on. Psychiatrists too try to form diagnoses, even though it can be difficult in their chosen field, and some argue that it is unhelpful. Psychiatric diagnosis is also less effective in its job of narrowing possibilities than in some other branches of medicine. This makes psychiatry one of the less precise specialties, with many uncertainties. In consequence, it can be easy for misunderstandings to arise between service users, their relatives and the psychiatric team.

Experiencing a severe mental illness

Schizophrenia is one of the most severe mental illnesses. It is seen all over the world with a similar frequency, in both modern and traditional societies. It cannot therefore be said that it is one of the burdens of modern civilisation. It is now thought to be somewhat more frequent in males than in females. In women, it often starts a few years later and has a somewhat better outlook. It is more common among people lower down the social scale, and we now think this may be the effect of social disadvantage as well as the result of sufferers doing less well in life than they might otherwise have done.

It might be best to start by saying what schizophrenia is not. It is not, despite what many people still seem to believe, a split personality of the Jekyll and Hyde type. There is no rapid switch from perfect normality to a totally different, often unpleasant, pattern of behaviour, so different it is as if the person has become someone else. Psychiatrists call this rather rare condition 'hysterical split personality', not schizophrenia.

Mental health professionals recognise schizophrenia mainly by the presence of delusions, hallucinations and other unusual experiences, such as the feeling of being followed. Delusions are unusual beliefs, 'mad ideas', while hallucinations often take the form of internal or external voices that others cannot hear. We describe these symptoms in more detail below.

The problems may start suddenly and dramatically, but often follow a gradual deterioration: the person may become less sociable and less able to study or work in a consistent way. They may become less affectionate, or suspicious, so that relatives find it hard to get through to them any more. In cases like this with a gradual onset, the definite features of schizophrenia may appear only after months or even years. This makes it difficult for mental health professionals to be sure what is happening, at least at the beginning.

Mary was an eighteen year old who developed schizophrenia. She still lived at home, and had always been a shy person. She was very close to her widowed father. She enjoyed quiet activities like fishing but would also go out to a pub or visit friends to listen to music. Over a period of some months, she felt less like going out. It made her feel very self-conscious, even a bit jittery. She did not really like the sense of being the centre of attention. However, she enjoyed the company of her friends, so she often invited them round. They were a bit boisterous and Mary was glad just to sit on the sidelines watching them. It made her feel safe. However, because they were noisy, the neighbours complained one night and her father was embarrassed, so she didn't ask them round again. She began to find that her usual activities were a real effort and, eventually, beyond her. Her elder brother came round one evening and dragged her out to a local pub. Mary did not want to go, and felt dreadful when she got there. She felt as if everyone was looking at her, that somehow they knew all about her and were talking about her. She made an excuse to leave as early as possible, but was still upset when she got home. The next evening something happened that made her feel even more frightened. While she was in her bedroom, she could hear people talking about her. There seemed no doubt about it, although when she looked out of the window and the door there was no-one around. Moreover, the voices, whoever they were, were not being very nice about her, using language and making suggestions that upset her. She kept very quiet about this for a couple of days. However, she began to have strange ideas that she could not stop thinking about, for instance, that she was pregnant. She thought she could feel the baby stirring inside of her. As she had never had sexual relations with anyone, she thought that she could only have been made pregnant by a spirit or a ghost, and the more she thought about this the more convinced she became. Finally Mary told her father what had been going on. He called their General Practitioner (GP).

This story gives an idea of what it was like for one person who developed what was diagnosed as schizophrenia. The experience differs in detail from case to case, but it is rarely anything but unpleasant. The experiences Mary had, together with some that she didn't, will be described further when we write about particular symptoms below. Remember, however, that what is a symptom to the doctor or relative is a very real and often very frightening experience to the person involved.

Fortunately Mary responded well to treatment and recovered completely, although she remained a rather shy and diffident young woman. Clearly, it would have been very difficult for anyone to be sure what was going on in the early stages of her mental health problems, or that it was anything more than 'just a phase'. Once the full picture emerged, however, there could be no doubt that Mary had had schizophrenia.

There are, in fact, two sorts of symptoms in schizophrenia. Hallucinations and delusions may be rather dramatic but aren't usually present all the time. However, the negative symptoms, described on page 35, can actually be more damaging. If someone with schizophrenia doesn't have any negative symptoms, he or she may be fairly well between attacks of the more dramatic symptoms. Some lucky people indeed may only have a single attack, and recover.

Simon was like this. He was a thirty-three year old married man who worked as an electrical engineer. He seemed to have been a cheerful and effective person before his illness. Following what appeared to be a minor problem at work, he suddenly became very frightened, and claimed that the local radio mast was controlling his brain. He was admitted to hospital where he was observed for a few days without being given any medication. His state of mind rapidly improved and after a few weeks he was able to take up his ordinary life again. So far he has not had any return of his upsetting thoughts.

What we call schizophrenia takes many forms, so it is hardly surprising that doctors often find it difficult to give exact guidance about the outlook, the benefits of particular treatments and so on.

The problems most commonly begin in early adulthood: two thirds of sufferers will have had their first attack by the time they are thirty. However, it can develop at any time of life, right up into old age.

Maude was a 71 year old woman who had followed a career in the civil service with some success. She was widowed and her children lived in the next town. Some time before, she had had a minor difference of opinion with her next door neighbour, and she became rather embarrassed whenever she met him as the problem had never really been resolved. This became worse, so that she would avoid his eye rather than say good morning. Not surprisingly, the neighbour was not sure how to respond to this snub and was rather embarrassed himself. Maude took this as indicating that he was ashamed of something, although she wasn't sure what. However, this gradually became clear to her: his shifty behaviour must be the result of something he was up to, and Maude reckoned that other little pieces of evidence confirmed that he was secretly making bombs for a terrorist group. This explained the rather unusual chemical smell she thought she could detect lingering about her own house and garden. Her children were never able to pick up this smell, and were surprised at her allegations about the neighbour whom they had always previously found rather pleasant. Nor were they convinced by her claim that his wife had been passing messages to fellow conspirators by the order in which she hung clothes on the washing line.

Schizophrenia is rare before adolescence, although it is not unknown. Sometimes it comes out of the blue. On the other hand, some people who develop schizophrenia have always had eccentric, quirky or solitary personalities: however, it must be said that most people like that do not develop schizophrenia.

Our ideas about mental illness have developed over a long period, mainly the last two hundred years. Ideas about schizophrenia began to crystallize at the end of the Nineteenth Century, when it came to be seen as a separate and identifiable condition with certain characteristic features. A distinction was particularly made between it and manic-depressive illness. Cases of the latter were grouped together because it was thought their central feature was a disorder of mood. Mood is a word for feelings like happiness, sadness, fear or anger. The idea of manic depressive illness was based on pulling together psychiatric conditions typified by two sorts of mood disturbance, namely depressed and elevated mood. While most people who suffer from episodes of elevated mood also experience episodes of depressed mood, the opposite is not true. As a result, the category of manic-depressive illness included many more people suffering only from attacks of severe depression than people who suffer from both. However, it was thought for much of the last century that there were important similarities that made it reasonable to include all cases within this one condition, manic depressive illness.

You may still hear the phrase manic-depressive illness, or hear someone described as a 'manic-depressive'. However, things have changed. It is now generally thought that the processes that underlie the condition in which people may be prone to both elevated and depressed mood are different from those in people who only suffer from episodes of depressed mood. These conditions are now termed bipolar and unipolar affective disorder (affective is an adjective that means mood-related, while polar refers to the two opposite ends of the condition, depression and elation).

Bipolar disorder (BPD) is one of the most serious mental health problems of adult life, although its impact is usually less devastating than schizophrenia. Like schizophrenia, it occurs throughout the world. It differs from unipolar depression in the way that it affects the sexes. While about twice as many women as men suffer from unipolar depression, the sexes are equally affected by bipolar disorder. Bipolar disorder is fairly rare, indeed, rarer than schizophrenia, whereas unipolar disorder is considerably more common (some people think it is becoming commoner). The bipolar type often begins in early adult life, whereas unipolar disorder is more likely to emerge as people get older.

However, the picture is even more complicated than this, as both bipolar and unipolar disorder can sometimes, but not always, be associated with psychotic symptoms like those seen in schizophrenia. Moreover, unipolar depression shades into states of unhappiness that may be completely understandable in terms of people's miserable circumstance, and are therefore, in a sense, normal. Thus the term depression is necessarily a loose one, being used to describe anything from normal unhappiness to those abnormal moods that seem to be the result of an illness, and it is true that it may sometimes be hard to draw the line. The mood disturbance in unipolar and bipolar affective disorder centres on happiness or sadness. However, it is far greater and more persistent than most of us normally experience. People are either hopelessly gloomy and miserable, looking at things in a very pessimistic light (depression) or wildly elated and energetic with big ideas about themselves and their abilities and a reduced need for sleep (mania). The most severe form of unipolar disorder is usually called major depressive disorder or major depressive episode.

However much clinicians may argue the finer points (and they do), an episode of affective disorder makes a disturbing experience.

Susan was a 24 year old teacher who had married about three years previously. She and her husband had moved to London where they had bought a pleasant modern flat. She worked in a local infant school. She liked the work, although she did have opinions about teaching that had led to minor disagreements with the headmistress. Working as an infant teacher is always strenuous, but Susan usually had energy to spare.

However, over a period of a few weeks, she felt as though the work was becoming too much for her. She felt really tired when she got home, and unable to devote herself to the preparations she normally made for the next day's teaching. She normally cooked the evening meal, something she did efficiently and almost automatically, but this too she found had become a real effort. She somehow got through her days but then lay around in the evening in an exhausted state. In the past, she and her husband had enjoyed going out together, but she now felt this to be completely beyond her: she made excuses and her husband fell in with this quieter life fairly amicably, feeling merely that she was going through a tough patch at school and would benefit from the rest. He was solicitous and tried to support and comfort her. One evening, although he worried that it might be a problem, he moved from being affectionate into trying to make love. This distressed Susan a lot although she attempted, not very successfully, to hide it. Not being able to respond sexually was bad enough, but she also felt completely out of touch with her normal affection for him, almost as if he was a stranger. She began to feel that a woman like that couldn't be much good and her sense of guilt became laceratingly painful. She became unable to think of anything except her painful preoccupation with herself and her feelings. She could hardly do anything and she felt slow, stupid and old. Her husband meanwhile was becoming increasingly and desperately worried about her. She still drove herself to go to work but one morning the burden became too much and she walked out of school and went home with out telling anyone. She phoned her husband who came home and called their family doctor.

Although at first it sounds quite similar, John's story is rather different. John was a little older than Susan, but he too became depressed over a period of weeks. He stayed at home and was visited by his family doctor who gave him antidepressant tablets. He seemed to be responding to this treatment and his doctor was pleased with his progress.

By this time, John felt pretty good and quite enthusiastic about going back to his work as a telephone engineer. He rang up his personnel officer to arrange this. He told his wife that, as he was completely recovered, there was not much point in staying at home. When he got to work on his first day back, a certain number of relatively easy tasks had been set aside for him. He completed these very quickly and without difficulty, and felt very pleased with the way things had gone. He was pleased also to see his workmates, and rapidly overcame their slight awkwardness at having him back after 'a bit of mental trouble'. In fact, as he was feeling quite jokey, he soon had them all laughing and relaxed. His manager was also glad to have him back so obviously recovered.

Over the next two days John became convinced that one particular working practice, which previously he had put up with as a bit of a chore, was in fact grossly inefficient. He thought out how things actually should be done, and saw what a major change for the better it would be if this change was brought in. He accordingly asked to see the manager who was somewhat taken aback when he found out why he had requested the interview. The manager raised a number of fairly obvious objections to John's proposal, although he acknowledged that it had some good points. John expounded his view fairly forcefully, and left feeling the manager was more stupid than he had thought. He did not, however, let this blight his day. When he returned from work, he told his wife all about it. In the evening he had a good idea. His car was almost due for a service. He would save himself money by doing it himself. He drove out and bought a large can of oil and returned to the garage where he carried out an oil change. Although he knew in principle how to do this, he had never done it before and made rather a mess. However, this was a minor consideration compared with the sense of satisfaction with which he returned, rather dirty, to the house. His wife looked unsure when he said he proposed to service the car on a regular basis, and he felt she was unadventurous and bit of a killjoy. She confirmed this opinion by going to bed at 11 o'clock. John didn't fancy sleeping just yet so he played some Mozart, music he had always been fond of. Tonight it seemed particularly pleasing. It was around 4.00 a.m. that the great idea struck him, no less than a completely new way of transmitting telephone messages. It was like a blinding light in its brilliant simplicity. He rummaged out a large and out of date diary and began to put his ideas on paper as he was terrified they would leave him before he could get them down. His wife found him still scribbling when she came down in the morning. He said he wasn't going to work as he had something important to work on at home. However, at 10.00 a.m. he went out and when he came back he told his wife that he had drawn money out of the bank to finance a business venture designed to develop and market his new telephone system. The enthusiastic and naive way in which he talked about this led her to call the GP. John was not pleased to see her, as he was feeling very good indeed. His experiences would be regarded as typical of a bipolar disorder.

There is no doubt from the descriptions above that depression is a very unpleasant experience indeed. Sometimes mania is too, as the person may feel very irritable and 'pressured'. However, as many people do, John actually felt good when he was in a manic state. This can pose real problems, particularly if people, while denying that they are unwell, do things they will later greatly regret. Getting them to cooperate in receiving help can then be very difficult indeed.

Unipolar and bipolar affective disorders typically come on in separate episodes, and people are usually fairly well in between. Episodes may develop over a few days in either type of disorder, but people with the unipolar condition often become depressed gradually, over a period of weeks or months.

Compared with physical illness, mental disorders do last quite a long time. Psychiatrists are used to this, but you may not be. However, things have improved. Before effective treatment was available for affective disorders, episodes might last from six months to two years, but nowadays six months is usually the maximum, and many episodes are considerably shorter. Episodes of bipolar disorder tend to be a bit shorter than in the unipolar version, but may occur more frequently.

Many people have only one attack of depression, but most do relapse. This may be after years of good health. Once a pattern of relapse has developed, the gap between episodes may tend to shorten, although this is not always the case. Some people may be persistently depressed, and this can cause great problems, as you will know if you live with them.

Negative symptoms (see page 35) do occur in bipolar disorder, but much less commonly than in schizophrenia. Sometimes it may be difficult for mental health professionals to decide whether someone is suffering from schizophrenia or bipolar disorder. The diagnosis is usually based on the most recent presentation, so it may not stay the same in different episodes. This is less worrying than it sounds, for in borderline cases treatment is determined by the features of the problem rather than by its particular label. Sometimes these intermediate disorders are called schizoaffective. They are treated rather like schizophrenia, but behave more like bipolar disorder, usually being episodic in nature, with recovery in between.

CAUSES

Despite years of effort and research, our knowledge of the origins of severe mental illness is still a long way from being complete. There is clearly no simple cause. We know that a whole range of factors are more common in those who suffer from it in its various forms. It is often suggested that these factors work together to produce psychiatric ill health. However, association does not necessarily mean cause, and even if there are causal links they may not be present in every individual sufferer. Moreover, the suspected causes may not be enough in themselves to lead to the development of psychiatric disorder. Thus there are people who seem to be subject to all the factors, but never become mentally ill. Equally, there are people who seem to have had none of the risk factors, but become unwell all the same. Over the last fifteen years, there have been a number of advances: these generally confirm that the causes of severe psychiatric illness are complicated, and also that the causes of different illnesses overlap.

Severe mental illness and genetic inheritance

It has been known for a very long time that most mental illnesses run in families. This is certainly true of both schizophrenia and bipolar disorder, to a roughly similar degree. Clear evidence for this comes from the study of twins. There are two sorts of twins, those that come from a single fertilized egg and those that come from two separate eggs. Twins of the first sort are genetically identical, that is, they share all the genetic instructions that determine our characteristics. Twins of the second type are really like ordinary brothers and sisters who happen to have been born at the same time; although they are closely related, on average they only share half their genetic instructions, so they are called non-identical twins. Take schizophrenia as an example. If it has a genetic part to its causation, you would expect the identical twin of someone with schizophrenia to have a much greater chance of developing the disorder than the non-identical twin of such a person. When groups of identical and of non-identical twins are compared, this is exactly what is found. It means that the tendency to these illnesses is at least partly 'built in'. This may worry people who suffer from the disorder, and their carers too: where one person is affected, there is a risk, usually fairly small, that other members of the family may also develop the same or similar problem. This is an important topic, so we discuss it at some length on page 64. It should be noted however that in 30–40% of cases where an identical twin has schizophrenia, their co-twin does not, so the condition cannot be wholly genetically determined.

A draft of the human genetic code was worked out in 2000, and was virtually complete by 2004. This has made it possible, at least in principle, to identify particular genes that may be associated with schizophrenia and bipolar disorder, both within families with several affected members, and in the population at large. At the time of writing, seven genes have been tentatively linked with schizophrenia and five with bipolar disorder. Interestingly, four of these genes are associated with both disorders: this suggests that some of the overlap in the symptoms of the two conditions comes about because of a genetic overlap. However, none of these genes seems to be associated with an increase in the rate of schizophrenia of more than about twofold. It is reasonable to suppose that someone with the misfortune to have several of these genes will have a greater risk of developing the condition than someone with a single gene, but this has not yet been demonstrated in practice. Moreover, finding a relevant gene does not yet tell us very much about how or why individuals are affected by it. Nor does it yet lead to new treatments, although it may do eventually.

Severe mental illness and the environment

The outside circumstances that affect us throughout our lives can be broadly separated into the physical and the social environment. A number of physical environmental factors have been implicated in the development of severe mental illness. Thus schizophrenia in particular may sometimes result from significant damage to the brain from various sources – what the medical profession in a nice piece of understatement calls a 'physical insult'.

One example of this is that complications and difficulties during pregnancy and at birth are more common in babies who as adults develop schizophrenia. Another is provided by the hunger winter in the Netherlands in 1944: children born just after this had an increased risk of schizophrenia, suggesting that malnourishment in pregnancy can affect the developing brain of the unborn baby. This implies that damage in the very early stages of life may result in a tendency to the condition, even though it does not appear until much later. We have only the most speculative ideas about how this delayed reaction might actually work. Head injury in childhood or adulthood may also sometimes be followed by schizophrenia. In a few instances, schizophrenia can follow another, physical, illness, such as epilepsy and certain uncommon bodily diseases. In most cases the connection is pretty clear because the physical condition produces its own symptoms by which it is readily recognised. Schizophrenia may also be linked to infection with certain viruses. However, while there is reasonable evidence for a degree of association between some types of viral infection and schizophrenia, it is unlikely to account for many cases. In the 1920s and 1930s, the viral epidemic of encephalitis lethargica did indeed result in several cases of schizophrenia (but also of other mental conditions). There is some evidence connecting influenza epidemics and schizophrenia: the children of mothers who were pregnant with them during one of these epidemics have an increased risk of developing schizophrenia. Other, non-viral, infections have been associated with the features both of schizophrenia and of manic depressive illness. The most famous of these was syphilis of the brain, otherwise known as General Paresis of the Insane (GPI). Although this played havoc among the Victorians, eminent and otherwise, it is now so rare that we have only seen a handful of cases in our professional lives and certainly none recently.

In general, recognisable physical causes for bipolar disorder are rather rare, but also occur. They are most often the result of physical diseases, for instance those associated with abnormalities of the endocrine glands, the glands that make hormones.

Another sort of physical environmental cause is exposure to street drugs, although the relationship between taking them and the development of severe mental illness is unclear and almost certainly complicated. Street drugs are taken precisely because they are mind altering, so in a way it is not surprising if they turn out to cause permanent change, or at least a permanent increase in vulnerability to mental disturbance. However, it is also possible that people with a susceptibility to severe mental illness are inclined to take street drugs more frequently, in much the same way that they are more likely to smoke. This may partly be due to the short term calming effect typical of some of these drugs.

There has certainly been considerable discussion recently in the press and on TV about the effects of cannabis on psychosis. Smoking cannabis appears to increase the risk of severe mental illness by three times. Heavy use of cannabis before the age of 18 seems particularly dangerous. As many teenagers in the UK do smoke cannabis, this can be a considerable source of worry to parents and others. Heavy cannabis smoking certainly makes it more likely that individuals will feel paranoid and suspicious of others, and it may cause hallucinations. These effects are usually temporary, but for some cannabis can trigger an unpleasant episode of psychosis. The danger seems to be greater in people who are for other reasons at increased risk of developing the disorder, for instance if they have a family history of the disorder. It is therefore particularly sensible for such individuals to reduce or cut out cannabis use.

Other street drugs have similar effects, in particular amphetamines and cocaine. These may provoke the onset of severe mental illness or uncover the propensity to attacks. They are linked with both schizophrenia and bipolar disorder. One not uncommon pattern is for episodes of bipolar disorder to become increasingly easy to provoke by the consumption of these stimulant drugs, indicated by the reduced dose needed to set off an attack. Opiate drugs such as heroin do not seem so clearly connected with psychotic symptoms.

The disorders associated with drugs in this way cannot really be distinguished from severe mental illness that is not linked with street drug use. Psychiatrists will sometimes describe an illness as a drug-induced psychosis. This can sometimes lead to rather sterile and occasionally dangerous arguments with their colleagues, and perhaps with service users and carers too, about whether the sufferer 'really' has schizophrenia. Sometimes the attack will seem to be the direct effect of drug use: it may occur very clearly just after a heavy session of crack (for instance) and get better very quickly. In such a case it may be reasonable to reserve judgement about whether there is something underlying going on. However, the disorder will often appear to take on a life of its own and recur without as much provocation as before. The danger is that if the psychosis is seen as the result of the wilful actions of sufferers, less sympathy will be offered and less effort will be made to ensure that they are persuaded of the need for treatment.

Excessive use of alcohol can also be associated with psychotic symptoms, although the picture is usually a little different from that seen in schizophrenia or bipolar disorder. There are two main scenarios. The first is called delirium tremens, which means, rather graphically, the 'shaking madness' and is the result of alcohol withdrawal. When people who are physically dependent on alcohol stop drinking altogether or greatly reduce their consumption, they experience withdrawal symptoms. These include anxiety and agitation, which go with the shakiness and probably account for some of it. However they sometimes also have visual and auditory hallucinations. Sufferers will either 'treat' these by starting to drink again, or the symptoms will wear off in a few days. This is different from the second type of psychosis associated with alcohol abuse. This happens to people who drink very heavily and pretty constantly for many years. They then start to hear voices, which are often very persistent, intrusive, unpleasant, and irritating. However, unlike people who suffer from schizophrenia, those with alcoholic hallucinosis often have good insight into them and do not think they are the voices of real people. The hallucinosis is very persistent and will last for months or years, even if the sufferer stops drinking entirely. Finally, many people who suffer from schizophrenia drink more than is good for them, without there being a connection between the alcohol intake and their mental symptoms. However, the alcohol consumption may make it harder for them to take part as effectively in treatment or rehabilitation.

There has also been considerable research into the possibility that diet or allergic processes lie behind the development of severe mental illness. This research has not been very productive and it must be concluded that if these factors do have any effect, it is only to a minor extent or in rare cases.

The second sort of environmental influence on severe mental illness comes from our existence as social beings. Most of us share the belief that the things that happen to us as a result of other people's actions can affect our mental state in good ways and in bad. We usually try to interpret the onset of mental disorder in terms of the various events we have experienced. Indeed, it is when mental health problems occur, as they sometimes do, without being preceded by an obvious stress that they become even more incomprehensible and upsetting for the people who suffer from them, and for their friends and relatives.

Research backs up the idea that mental conditions, including schizophrenia and bipolar disorder, are often influenced by the stresses and strains of everyday living. Such stresses can take the form of some sudden misfortune or change in living circumstances, or of more enduring difficulties. Problems that most people manage to cope with seem to be able to push others into mental ill health, one assumes because of some kind of pre-existing tendency that way. However, there is also accumulating evidence that severely traumatic events and circumstances can lead to psychotic symptoms in quite a high proportion of people experiencing them. Examples include war trauma and child sexual abuse.

The last of these raises the question of whether childhood circumstances are generally associated with severe mental disorders. There seems little doubt that childhood is a more vulnerable time than we once thought. There is now quite good evidence that severely adverse circumstances and experiences in childhood are associated with a considerably increased risk of all forms of mental illness when people have grown up. While there could be many explanations for this, some of the link may be direct, arising because bad early experiences genuinely predispose towards the development of a vulnerability to mental problems at a later stage in life. These circumstances include physical and sexual abuse, and being brought up in local authority care or in a children's home. The disorders that follow such experiences certainly include schizophrenia and other psychoses, although we are unable to explain very well why the associated disorders take different forms in different people.

Fifty years ago a number of psychiatrists and psychologists believed strongly that schizophrenia arose directly out of an abnormal family environment in childhood. The best known proponent of this idea in Britain was the late R.D. Laing. The research on this at the time was never very good, and is now discounted. It did have the frequent and unproductive effect of making the unhappy parents of those who later developed schizophrenia feel both guilty and defensive. Because at the time mental health professionals were taught about this during their training, it also had a pervasive and unfortunate influence in making their attitudes towards the parents of people with schizophrenia rather punitive. Clinicians often behaved as though the parents were to blame, as though they had wilfully set out to behave in such a bad way towards their children that severe mental illness was virtually the inevitable consequence of these deliberate actions. Such attitudes are fortunately pretty rare now.

It is well established that people with schizophrenia are affected by tensions at home, but this is not very surprising and is hardly grounds for blaming parents. A similar effect has been found in bipolar disorder. These findings do carry the hope that relatives may be able to change things for the benefit of the sufferer, once they know how they might do this, and this is discussed further on p ( ).

Personality and the tendency to develop severe mental ill health
Personality is a mixture of the temperament you are born with and the effects of subsequent experiences. Between them, these are thought to limit our responses to the demands of our lives, so that the way we deal with particular situations may be recognised by our friends and relatives as being in some way typical of us. Each person's personality is a complex brew of various characteristics on which they differ from other people only in degree. The idea behind

personality is that it is rather unchanging throughout our lives. Indeed we may want to change it and find it beyond us. People whose personality seems particularly unusual may be described as having a personality disorder, although normal personality types shade into personality disorders very gradually, so it is very difficult to say when the border is crossed into something that might usefully be seen as a disorder.

The risk that someone will develop a severe mental health problem may be increased if they have a particular type of personality. Attempts have been made to link schizophrenia with a particular personality type, the schizoid personality. Such people are aloof, sensitive, solitary and not good at making emotional contact. However, there are many people like this who never develop schizophrenia. People who behave increasingly like this may indeed be showing the first signs of schizophrenia, but that is a rather different matter.

Another type of personality that is more securely linked with schizophrenia is the schizotypal personality. This shares the qualities of aloofness and eccentricity seen in schizoid personality, along with difficulties in maintaining relationships. However, there are also other traits, some of which are very common, affecting up to 30% of us. Such people are more likely to have unusual experiences, or odd ideas, and may even look out for them, finding them interesting. They can be rather suspicious and paranoid. They may occasionally experience unusual perceptions: voices, visions and odd bodily experiences. They may be quite obsessed with these experiences and are likely to find them positive. They thus do not generally tend to ask for help.

A small proportion of people with these experiences does find them distressing, or behaves in ways that distress others. As a result they are much more likely to contact mental health services. Our current understanding is that it is not just having unusual experiences that causes problems, but how we make sense of them. If you think you can hear the voice of God and find it comforting, you might not think of it as a problem. If you worry that the voice might be your neighbour, but are able to dismiss it as unlikely, you will still be relatively unlikely to need or ask for help. However if you decide the voice is to do with your neighbour persecuting you, and start complaining about him, that will often result in the involvement of mental health professionals and the diagnosis of mental illness.

A number of personality types have been implicated in bipolar disorder. One is the 'cyclothymic' personality – people like this are moody, in the sense that sometimes they are energetic and enthusiastic and sometimes gloomy and lethargic. It is possible that this personality type represents minor degrees of the mood swings that, if fully developed, would be called bipolar illness. It is thus not surprising that people with it sometimes make the move into a fully fledged illness. However, people who are persistently energetic and cheerful sometimes do surprise us by developing a 'nervous breakdown' – 'they're the last person you would have expected to have one'. This is the hypomanic personality, and people like that do indeed sometimes develop a severe depressive illness. Because those around them may be slow to recognise it, they may sometimes kill themselves before anyone realises the danger.

Another type of personality that often goes with a tendency to develop depressive illnesses is actually called the depressive personality. Some of this is probably the result of innate temperament, but people with this personality are most noticeable on account of their rather gloomy attitudes, which they have probably learned from their previous experience of life. They have a distorted view of themselves and the world which means that any new experience is interpreted in a gloomy and hopeless way. For such people, nothing good can ever happen because it if did, they wouldn't notice it or would find some way of devaluing it.

Finally, some people who are prone to depression are very obsessive and perfectionist. Because nothing is good enough for them, they can never feel good about things they have done. For most of us 'nobody's perfect' is a solace, for them it is a reproach.

In all probability, little can be done about basic temperament. However, more recently therapists have made successful attempts to change the attitudes and behaviour of individuals with persistently negative ways of thinking using the techniques of cognitive therapy (see page 131).

The bodily basis of severe mental illness
The evidence is now strong that both schizophrenia and bipolar disorder are associated with changes in various transmitter substances in the brain. The nerve cells in the brain form a sort of network, and work by switching each other on and off, a little bit like the switches in a computer (except they are analogue, not digital). One cell helps to

switch on the next in line by giving out a chemical compound, or transmitter substance. The brain uses a range of these substances in different places and if they are not being released in the right quantities, it is believed that mental health difficulties can follow. We are even in a position to make reasonable guesses about which transmitters, and where. Quite a lot of evidence for instance suggests that in schizophrenia there is some abnormality in the handling of the transmitter substance dopamine, particularly in the connections between the deeper parts of the brain and the areas nearer the surface (the 'cerebral cortex') where the more intellectual functions of the mind, such as perception, thought and judgement, are carried out. In crude terms, it is as if there is too much dopamine around. Drugs that suppress the action of dopamine also improve the clinical condition of someone with acute symptoms of schizophrenia.

Nowadays it is generally agreed that the dopamine theory does not account for all the features of schizophrenia. For instance, it is difficult to explain why schizophrenia typically does not arise in childhood or early adolescence. More elaborate theories suggest that the dopamine abnormality arises as the long-term effect of an earlier disturbance in nerve cells that use glutamate as a transmitter substance. These are located in a part of the underside of the brain called the hippocampus, and may be damaged or caused to malfunction either before the individual was born or in early childhood.

Another biological influence on these severe mental illnesses is exerted by the body's hormonal state. Some authorities have tried to explain the greater frequency of depression in women in terms of the action of the sex hormones. It used to be thought that the menopause was associated with an increase in depressive illnesses in women. This has recently been shown not to be true – women as a group are actually less depressed after the menopause. The hormonal changes brought about by childbirth are more important. These can lead to the so-called post partum ('after delivery') psychoses, which can take the form of schizophrenia or, more often, of bipolar disorder, but often show features of both. It is relatively rare, occurring after only one pregnancy in 500. Individuals rarely show negative symptoms (see page 35), and there is usually a good outcome. Further episodes occur following about one in five subsequent deliveries, and about half have later episodes that do not follow delivery. Hormones may also play a part in postnatal depression, a much milder, though still unpleasant, condition. There are however almost certainly social and psychological influences on this as well. There is a special Association for Post Natal Illness.

The best evidence for a hormonal explanation of depressive disorder actually concerns the stress hormone cortisol. The control of this hormone and its effects does not seem to be associated with gender, so this hormonal theory cannot explain why women are more prone to depression than men.

This summary of our knowledge about the causes of severe mental ill health may lead you to think that the enormous effort put into research has not reaped much in the way of reward. This is not strictly true. We think that the slow progress has come about because these conditions are actually extremely complex and subtle. Because of this, it seems rather unlikely that there will be any sudden breakthrough: research will find the answers gradually by piecing together what is almost certainly a very complicated jigsaw.

The prevalent view currently is that there is a complex chain of cause and effect, with one abnormality leading to another. The end of this chain is the emergence of severe mental disorder. Genes are potentially the starting point of the chain, but genes are actually directly responsible only for the production of proteins. They are therefore a long way from the subtle interaction between people's behaviour and environment that is the expression, for instance, of psychosis. Genes may be closer to abnormalities of brain function, for example, certain types of memory and recognition. These in turn may predispose people to misinterpret the world around them in various ways. This may encourage a downward spiral into beliefs and actions that eventually lead to a diagnosis of psychosis. At every level there are likely to be several factors, for example genes or abnormalities in psychological function, which interact with each other and also with factors at different levels. However, it is quite possible for earlier bits of the chain to be absent in individual sufferers. It is also possible for some of the cause and effect links to work in a direction opposite to what you might expect. It has been found for instance that particular environmental conditions may be required before certain genes work at all. In the wrong sort of environment, it is as if the gene did not actually exist. However, once the gene has been induced by environmental circumstances, it may be expressed even when those conditions no longer apply.

If we are right in thinking the causes of severe mental illness have this degree of complexity, it almost certainly follows that treatments are likely to be equally complicated. We shall see that this is so.

OUTLOOK

Is there a cure for mental illness? In view of the sheer complexity of the possible causes and the way they interact, you will not be too surprised to know that there is no clear answer to this question either. There is certainly no single effective cure for the conditions we have been talking about, but then this is also true of chronic medical problems like rheumatoid arthritis, asthma or cancer. However, there are different sorts of treatment available that together can help relieve both schizophrenia and bipolar disorder, either wholly or in part. Treatment may take the form of tablets (medication), individual therapy aimed at helping the person to understand and manage their problems better, the arrangement of the person's life in less stressful and more productive patterns, or family work to help carers cope more effectively with difficulties. Selecting the best combination of such treatments is often a subtle business that takes much thought on the part of the health professionals involved. We will take you through these issues at much greater length in chapter 4.

As we have suggested already, the outlook for mental illness varies: some attacks last for days, weeks or months; others, years or a lifetime. Even in the most prolonged conditions, there are variations in severity, and periods when the sufferer is relatively well.

People who have suffered an episode of mania or depression usually get better, although as many as 10% of those with the more severe forms do not. Although they may never have another episode, most will do so, usually after some years. Some, perhaps as many as 25%, may have minor mood swings between episodes which can impair their ability to function. Episodes which come on gradually are likely to improve relatively slowly, and a disorder that begins in later life does not have such a good outlook.

In general, the prospect for schizophrenia is less promising, but even here perhaps 20% experience only a single episode from which they recover. Even when we wrote the first edition of this book, only one person in ten was still in hospital five years after a first episode of schizophrenia. Very few now live in hospital, and most who would previously have done so are now in hostels and high support homes. However, while about half the people who develop an episode of schizophrenia recover, a large proportion may continue to have difficulties, usually not doing so well in life as they otherwise might. By difficulties we mean that the person is unable to do enough – looking after themselves, working, socialising – to make as full and as happy a life as they might have done otherwise. Around 10% will need round the clock care in some setting, not being able to manage on their own. The employment prospects for people with schizophrenia in Britain are much worse than they ought to be, given that a fair percentage has relatively little in the way of disability – only 10-15% are in employment.

The prospect for schizophrenia is better for those who do not have a previous family history. A relatively abrupt onset to the problem is (surprisingly) also a good sign, particularly if it followed some kind of sudden stress. Negative symptoms (see page 35) indicate a poorer outlook, mainly because they will probably persist when acute symptoms have gone, and are more difficult to improve.

From what we have said above, you will gather that it is not really possible at the beginning of a severe mental illness to predict what is going to happen later on. Professionals frequently avoid forthright opinions at this stage, mainly because they are worried that what they say may turn out later to have been misleadingly optimistic or pessimistic. Your relative will be offered various treatments, and these will affect the outcome in various ways and to a varying extent. Obviously, their circumstances, their own reactions, and their ability to manage will influence the success of any treatment they are given. Considerable time may be needed, and it can be months or even years before improvements become apparent and are stable. All psychiatric professionals work within this sort of time span. It can be confusing and unnerving for you and your relative to find that, unlike in physical illness, rapid improvements may not be expected.

SYMPTOMS

We are now going to take you through the symptoms of schizophrenia and bipolar disorder.

Many of these you may immediately recognise from your experiences of your relative's behaviour. Others you will not know about, but we think it is useful to learn what can happen to people's behaviour as a result of mental ill health and to avoid being caught unawares by new developments. We will concentrate particularly on those symptoms that are distressing, confusing or frequent.

Mental illness often shows itself through changes in mood even when this is not the central feature of the disorder. Normally most of us keep on a fairly even keel, although sometimes we may feel especially happy or a bit fed up. The mood of people with mental illness can be much more extreme than most of us ever experience.

People can be said to be depressed in mood when they remain sad, miserable, mournful or gloomy for days or weeks at a time, and when this mood persists despite all the efforts of themselves and those around them. One of the most characteristic symptoms is that the sufferer can no longer take pleasure in anything at all. Depressed people feel pessimistic and hopeless about themselves and the world, often blaming themselves for things that go wrong. They withdraw into themselves and don't talk much. Their energy goes, they are easily tired and they let things slide. In general, they cannot be bothered with things any more, and often lose interest in sex. They may feel so worthless that there is nothing left but to end things as quickly as possible, by an overdose or in a more violent manner. Those who do intend suicide will usually give some warning (see page 52).

In some people the loss of energy is very marked indeed. They move more slowly than they normally do, and often complain that they are walking as though they were twenty or thirty years older than they actually are. Sometimes, they may stop moving much at all, staying in bed most of the time.

Some depressed people in contrast become very agitated. They cannot keep still and often pace from room to room wringing their hands. They may continually ask their relatives and friends for reassurance – 'I'm not going mad, am I?' 'It will be all right, won't it?' This distress is painful to see and, if you have seen it, you will know that at the same time it can be extremely wearing.

Disturbed sleep is common in the mentally ill. Some people have trouble getting off to sleep, often because of depressing or worrying thoughts. Others sleep fitfully and restlessly. Some depressed people wake up in the early hours of the morning, a time they often feel at their worst. They lie there in anguish, feeling crushed beneath the weight of their sorrows. Those with mania in contrast frequently manage with very little sleep, remaining very energetic into the small hours, and likewise waking early and refreshed. People who have been mentally ill for some time occasionally develop odd ways of living, waking at night and sleeping by day. This is often part of a general tendency to avoid people.

Because depression makes people feel physically run down, they sometimes do not realise they are depressed, but think they must have some physical disease. Ordinary aches and pains become more noticeable. This may come out as fears of cancer or AIDS or venereal disease, and occasionally leads to a preoccupation with physical health that can end up being very tiresome for relatives. Because bodily aspects are emphasised, the family doctor may not at first recognise the depression underlying the complaints, and may embark on unwarranted investigations and treatment. This mistake is easily made, and not uncommon.

Margaret was a middle aged woman who began to feel run down. At first she put this down to the fact that she was not as young as she used to be. She had always been a fastidious person of orderly habits, and she took more notice of an increasing tendency in herself to be constipated than other people might. What she didn't realise was that constipation is not uncommon in depression, part of the general slowing that happens in moderately severe cases. She became very preoccupied with her bowels, so much so that she could not be bothered to go out socially any more. She began to notice pains in her stomach. She visited her family doctor who prescribed a laxative, without much effect. Her appetite declined. At this point, she read a newspaper story about a television star who had died of cancer. She didn't tell anyone about this, but gradually came to the fearful realisation that her own symptoms were probably the result of cancer of the bowel. She was overwhelmed with anxiety which she bottled up for some time until at last she brought herself to return to her doctor. He took her seriously and referred her for investigations. This time he spotted that she was depressed, but thought it was a natural reaction to her fear of cancer. The investigations proved negative and the gastroenterologist thought she was greatly exaggerating her symptoms, so he referred her to a psychiatrist colleague. She was fortunately able to identify the true nature of Margaret's problem.

In contrast, some mentally ill people become 'high"; what the mental health professionals call hypomanic or manic. This is what happened to John (see p...). They are full of energy and ideas, and talk quickly and wittily. They race about getting things done (some of which are useful, some not). They may be found cleaning the cooker at 4 am, or may wake up the family at a similar time for an unplanned trip to the country. There is a danger they may seriously exhaust themselves (in the past, before effective treatment, such people sometimes actually died of exhaustion). They may get very irritable with those around them who try to impose a limit on their activity and their wild schemes. They are often what a psychiatrist might call disinhibited – if they feel like doing or saying something, they will do so, without regard for consequences. This may be very hurtful. They frequently make new relationships, sometimes sexual, with people they would not normally make friends with. A few people swing wildly from depression to elation in a manner that is very difficult to cope with indeed.

Some people may lose their emotional responses through mental ill health, becoming wooden and unreactive, however hard you try to get through to them. This can happen with depression, when someone is so frozen in their depressed mood that nothing seems to touch them. However, it is not uncommon in schizophrenia as well. People's faces usually show a constantly changing pattern of emotions and expressions, something so normal we don't even think about it until we are surprised by its absence. However, in a few cases of schizophrenia (and in some cases of problems affecting older adults such as dementia and Parkinson's disease), the facial expression is relatively fixed. This is unsettling. We feel unable to get through to the person any more, and they seem very unrewarding to be with, so much do we rely on facial expression for the feeling of being in contact with the other person. This symptom has become less common since people have been managed in the community for longer periods.

Normally it is possible to have an effect on someone else's mood. In particular, we can usually cheer up friends and relatives who are feeling down. One of the upsetting things about the change in mood that occurs in mental illness is that it does not seem to respond to our efforts, and certainly not to those of the person with these difficulties.

Another of the symptoms of severe mental illness is a belief in things that seem wildly improbable or impossible. Other people's arguments do not shift these strongly held convictions. Unusual beliefs of this sort are called delusions, and sufferers who act on them may get into a lot of difficulty and trouble with those around them. The most common belief is of being persecuted, perhaps even by members of their own family. This may lead to arguments, and even fights. One man thought that terrorists were leaving cars parked in particular places as a signal to him that they were going to attack him. Others, especially those who are manic, may have unrealistically big ideas about themselves and their abilities. This may lead them to spend money carelessly or to develop grand schemes. They may even be able to persuade other people to take part in them. One man obtained a £20,000 loan from his ordinarily hard-headed bank manager to finance a completely unrealistic business scheme.

Depressed people may be preoccupied with some imaginary wrong they have done, feeling horribly guilty. One elderly woman thought that she might have allowed a cannabis plant to grow in her garden and the police were coming to take her away for trial and inevitable execution. Others may develop ideas that they are riddled with cancer or venereal disease.

People who have had delusions for some time may realise that others quite obviously do not share their ideas. They may then keep quiet, which reduces further any likelihood that they might discuss alternative views. Delusions may still make their behaviour unpredictable and hard to understand even if they don't talk about them. Some advice on coping with delusional ideas is given on page 44.

Many people with schizophrenia and some of those with bipolar disorder will hear things that others cannot, often voices talking about them. Their thoughts and ideas are no longer understood as internal and private, but experienced as coming from outside. These experiences are real, what is different about them is that they are misattributed: understood as coming from an external source. Often such voices are upsetting. People hearing them may react in a seemingly strange or violent way. They may shout back at the voices, go round to sort out the neighbours they think are making comments about them, or make complaints at the local police station. Hearing voices like this is usually most unpleasant. Many people describe feeling very frightened, powerless and not in control. Others get used to them, and for some they provide comfort and company. Often such voices discuss areas of genuine concern, even if they are distorted, or recognised as 'the devil' or 'my neighbour'. It used to be thought that hearing voices was itself a sign of a severe mental illness, but it is now known that such experiences are not uncommon. A surprisingly large proportion of the general population has sometimes heard disembodied voices, but in most cases the experience is fleeting and has very little impact. We now think it is the meaning, the distress and the problems associated with such experiences that determine whether they are seen as symptoms of mental ill health. In our view the most important part of this is whether the voice is understood as part of your own thinking, even if it is heard outside your head. If a voice can be understood as part of your own thinking, although experienced in a different way, like a memory, or a dream, then it can be rationalised and will not be so frightening. The technical term for such voices is auditory hallucinations.

Hallucinations may also be of things seen, although this is less common. One man had visions of choirs of angels when he became manic, but when he was depressed he saw the most dreadful and excruciating torments of hell. Other peple may smell or taste things that no one else can. People experiencing such hallucinations may accuse relatives, neighbours or friends of trying to gas or poison them. One woman was convinced that the man in the flat above had built a pipe into her wall and was passing a lethal gas into her sitting room.

People may sometimes have hallucinations of touch. One woman felt hands going around her neck to strangle her as she walked down the street. Sometimes she would have some insight into this and be able to tell herself that it was just an odd experience, it was not really happening to her. At other times, the power of the hallucination completely convinced her of its reality. This was very terrifying indeed, as you might imagine; she felt she was about to die and there was nothing she or anyone else could do about it. Other hallucinations may have a sexual aspect: people may occasionally claim they have a phantom lover, or say 'a demon visits me at night' because of strange and unprovoked sexual sensations.

People with psychosis sometimes have other odd experiences. They may experience unusual changes in their own thinking. They

may fe
their ow
what they
stop, leavi
completely e
away their tho
They may also
belong to them, t
inserted or droppe
a pool. Others may
control what they are
had half of his brain on
and actions. Another man
into his brain so that MI6

Some of these experience   e hard
to have any idea what it mus   s again can
isolate those experiencing ther   , and can add to
feelings of being stigmatised an   ood.

Schizophrenia and mania can   affect the ability to think straight in a sometimes spectacular way. The connection between thoughts becomes much less obvious, so the sufferer jumps from topic to topic in an unpredictable way. This usually reveals itself in disjointed speech. In mania, it may still be possible to follow the connections, even though they might be ones we would never think of ourselves. Occasionally there appears to be no connection at all between sentences, and in extreme cases the link between words in the same sentence may also vanish. This makes the sufferer's speech incomprehensible, as might be imagined. Disordered speech is most common in acute episodes of psychosis.

One thing you may worry about particularly in connection with a friend or relative with severe mental illness is the question of violent behaviour. People with a severe mental illness are, as a group, only slightly more prone to violence than the rest of the population. This certainly does not apply to everyone with mental health problems, as mental illness often makes people withdraw from friends and relatives and become apathetic. They are then much less likely to be violent at all. However, some people do behave violently while they are ill, and such violence is disturbing, as it is often unforeseen. There are four broad types of violence.

The first can arise from increased irritability – they may be on a

s understandable, but is an
Such violence can be avoided if
that it may occur, notice when it is
k as a result. It is likely to happen when
mething your relative asks for, or disagree with
says.

econd type, the person strikes out unexpectedly at
he nearby. Afterwards, it is possible to see that the violent
tion was indeed provoked by the other person's action, but only
because it was misinterpreted. It could not have been anticipated
that their behaviour would be so provocative. One man, Alan, had
become preoccupied with the belief that his body was changing sex.
A friend commented in a friendly way that he seemed to have put
on a bit of weight recently, and was surprised when Alan struck him.
Alan had taken the comment as a confirmation of his worst fears.

The third type of violence, too, is often unpredictable, although
fortunately much rarer than those described above. This arises
because the perpetrator experiences command hallucinations. These
are what they sound like, that is, hallucinations that order the
sufferer to do something. They are experienced as very forceful
indeed so the person finds them very frightening and almost
impossible to resist. Sometimes people experiencing these will tell
someone about them – their relatives, their doctor, their community
psychiatric nurse. If they are being told to do something violent, this
information needs to be communicated so the risk can be
minimised. Some people have committed murder under the
influence of command hallucinations.

The fourth type of violence is also rare. It is planned by the
sufferer, but arises because of delusional beliefs about his or her
circumstances, and so is extremely difficult to predict. Sometimes
the person gives warning, and obviously such warnings should
again be taken very seriously.

One man with schizophrenia had delusions of persecution,
feeling that people were out to harm him. He kept these ideas to
himself and his family was astonished when he made a murderous
attack on a favourite uncle. It later turned out that he suspected his
uncle of orchestrating the whole campaign against him.

Violent and murderous behaviour by people with schizophrenia
has been the subject of exaggerated media interest. A well known
example is Christopher Clunes who murdered Jonathan Zito at a

tube station. While this was an appalling tragedy for the victim and the victim's family, and indeed the perpetrator as well, it should be emphasized that such murders have not become more common, occurring in Britain at a consistent rate of around 20 per year for the last 25 years. This is over a period when the general homicide rate has gradually risen, so the proportion committed by people with mental disorder has actually fallen.

Depressed people occasionally take sudden and unexpected violent actions. What usually happens is that the depression is so deep that sufferers see no future for themselves or their immediate family. Such people may kill relatives from a misplaced sense of pity. The newspapers occasionally carry stories of a mother or father who has murdered all their children and then killed themselves. Such tragedies are fortunately quite rare. They serve to illustrate that violence is sometimes a possibility when judgement is impaired by mental illness. Violence is always difficult to cope with, but we have provided some guidelines on page 56, in the hope that they will help those of you who are faced with it.

Some of the most difficult symptoms for relatives to come to terms with are the so-called 'negative' symptoms. People who for some years have had severe mental health problems (especially schizophrenia), 'lose' bits of their normal behaviour. They cannot concentrate for long, they lose interest, they have no energy. One mother said 'she's lost her spark". Individuals may sit around listlessly, watching television, though taking in very little. They may lie in bed for long periods and avoid people. They may stop looking after themselves, becoming untidy and rather careless about personal hygiene. Sometimes table manners may deteriorate and other social graces may vanish. They lose the ability to react emotionally, appearing thoughtless towards people they used to be close to. They may seem to be less intelligent than before. At the same time they become stubborn. All in all, these so-called negative symptoms, almost invariably the consequence of prolonged schizophrenia, are amongst the most difficult problems for relatives. This is partly because it is quite hard to see them as resulting from a disorder, rather than laziness, lack of feeling or even sheer bloody-mindedness. Fortunately, the worst sorts of negative symptoms have become much rarer following the introduction of community care.

Most people with mental ill health are quite aware that something is wrong with the way they think and feel. However, in the more severe conditions, insight can be lost. Sufferers cannot see that their beliefs are unbelievable, and they may express the oddest ideas with considerable vehemence. If your relative is like this, you may sometimes have found yourself being steered into arguing with them, although you probably realized that this was quite pointless. However, when the belief is merely improbable (a person in London feeling they are under constant surveillance by MI5), relatives may occasionally find themselves wondering if there might not be some truth in what they say. Sometimes, if they are easily swayed, they may even act as if they too believe what the suffer claims. One rather shy young man developed a severe depressive illness in which he believed that he had committed a rape on a girl he had talked to on a couple of occasions about ten years previously. He thought the police were going to come for him and kill him. He managed to persuade his mother, with whom he lived, that this might be true. The desk sergeant at the local police station was surprised to receive a call from her, asking to speak to 'George the exterminator'. We will discuss how to cope with delusional ideas on page 44.

2 Coping with Severe Mental Illness

THE PROBLEMS YOU MAY HAVE TO DEAL WITH

Some of you will be fortunate: your relative will recover and the family will gradually get over the turmoil. If this does not happen or if your relative recovers but symptoms return, then living with them may give rise to a variety of problems. As well as all the ordinary difficulties that families may face, there are extra ones, often unrecognised or poorly understood, that arise as a result of severe mental illness. The modern developments in community care mean families are now expected to cope at home at an earlier stage of a disorder than was the case 40 years ago. The average mental hospital stay is now around three weeks, and almost all patients are discharged within a year. Many services now try to offer 'home treatment' where the person is never admitted to hospital, but lives at home all the time.

Relatives often want to be involved in assisting recovery, and in providing continuing support if this is needed. In the past, relatives often felt that they themselves did not receive assistance, that their requests for advice were ignored and that their problems were not considered until a crisis emerged. Unfortunately, a recent survey (2004) confirms that many carers still feel the same. Historically mental health professionals used to see relatives as part of the environment of their client, rather than as people with needs of their own. In the last decade, changes such as the Community Care Act of 1992 specified that carers should be consulted and included in care plans. This has been consolidated into guidelines such as the National Service Framework for Mental Health (1999). These changes have aimed to ensure that carers should be more visible to care planners, and that they should be seen as people with needs of their own, separate from patients' needs. However, despite the legislation, it is difficult for carers to access decision making, and to feel their voices can be heard. Organisations such as RETHINK (see Appendix) continue to try to change this.

RECOVERY

There is still considerable confusion between problems caused by an episode, and its possible unseen after-effects, and those caused by other factors, such as the individual's character and own reaction to what has happened, or the effects of medication. Because of this, it can be extremely difficult for you to get the balance right. For instance it can be difficult to judge whether you are expecting too much of your relative or not expecting enough. Similarly, unreasonable behaviour should not be encouraged, but blaming your relative for behaviour that they cannot control will not be helpful either.

For instance in one family, one son, John aged 21, had developed psychosis, and it was very difficult for the other members of the family, mother, successfully working brother and step-father, to know what to expect. He had already changed from an active teenager with a talent for art, into someone who was suspicious, sometimes violent, and very unwilling to get out of bed. When some of the more dramatic symptoms got better in hospital and he returned home, he was still very uninterested in doing anything, difficult to talk to, and liable to lie in bed all day. The family tended to think that he had been prescribed too much medication, which meant they were angry with the hospital, or they thought he was just lazy, and got very angry at him. In fact some of the loss of interest and tiredness was not due to medication or personality but to the fact of having had an episode of psychosis. This is very common. However, it took a long time for the family to realise this, and to understand that, although John was responsible for some of his behaviour, some of it was beyond his control and he needed time and encouragement to become more active and more like his old self. In fact it took about a year and a lot of family effort for him to re-establish a routine and get himself a part-time job. Even then he still felt tired and had trouble concentrating sometimes.

This is a complex issue and it often takes time to make the right adjustments. It may be a considerable while, as in John's case, before some people regain their former interest in the outside world. Indeed, a few never seem to do this.

One mother lived with her 30 year old daughter Rachel. She had been very worried at the changes in her daughter, as Rachel had a particular idea that she looked unacceptable to the outside world, and refused to go out. With hospital admission and treatment this idea faded, and Rachel returned home and was able to go out with her mother. However she seemed to have lost her enthusiasm and spontaneity, and unless her mother made suggestions would stay indoors doing very little all day. After some months some of her interest came back, but it was a very gradual process.

A relative who has had a severe mental illness may also show much less in the way of facial expression and affection for the family and will be harder to talk to. This can be both confusing and hurtful; it need not mean that your relative feels less deeply, just that it is not expressed in the same open way. One father described it as 'you never know what they're thinking. He sits there all day and you'd think he'd be bored; he doesn't seem to be, but he never says'.

In this family the son, while retaining some odd ideas about others disliking him, was able to go to a day centre, but was rather uncommunicative most of the time. He would accept food and having his laundry done for him, but answered in monosyllables and never expressed gratitude or seemed at all curious about his parents' viewpoint, or how they might have been upset about his illness. This was understandably hurtful, and difficult for them to get used to.

Another problem is unpredictability. There may be some days when a person is 'her old self' and then quite suddenly 'I've lost her again'. These mood changes may occur without warning, so that an ordinary conversation can turn into a sudden series of accusations without apparent reason. Severe mental illnesses can affect people like this, and the sufferer is often not in control of these strong feelings that suddenly become convictions. It is usually best to be aware that this can happen and recognise it when it does. You should not feel that you have caused this switch of mood yourself.

The best strategy in this circumstance is normally to change the subject, distract your relative or leave them alone for a while. One family, whenever their daughter started a tirade against 'the Russians' would offer to make a cup of tea instead of pursuing an argument.

The after-effects of a severe mental illness can include loss of energy, sleeping a lot, spending time doing nothing and wanting to avoid people. Although it may look like it, you should not be tempted to see this just as laziness and unfriendliness but try to understand that it is an after effect. If someone does nothing else at all but sit in their room, this can be harmful. In such cases, your relative should be encouraged to go out, to join in with some other family activities (even if they say nothing), to do a short educational or leisure course, or attend a day or drop-in centre. It is not surprising if they spend a certain amount of time on their own, even if they appear completely unoccupied, and other family members should intrude on this gently. It is probably best to encourage them to participate, and to help with some household jobs, without demanding that they be done instantly or expecting too high a standard. Expectations can be gradually increased as competence and interest return.

Sometimes a lack of energy and a reluctance to be with people may lead some people with mental illness just to stay in bed. Relatives often find this difficult to deal with, being uncertain of the right approach. One mother found it useful and effective to offer cups of tea at regular intervals, together with a time check. She did not bring her daughter's breakfast, which remained on the table downstairs. Another mother adopted a more active approach. After calling her son several times, she would then go into his room if he had not got up by midmorning. She would laughingly ask: 'Head first or feet first?' and then physically pull his feet out of bed. He would then begin to get dressed.

UNACCEPTABLE OR EMBARRASSING BEHAVIOUR

While families vary in their tolerance, there are several sorts of behaviour they are likely to find unacceptable. For example, your relative may shout, swear or talk to themselves in a rather obvious manner, damage furniture or other objects, or threaten to harm themselves or others. Obviously, you will want this kind of behaviour to diminish, but you may feel unsure about the best way to do this without causing worse arguments or upsetting your relative. You may feel that you get no advice on this problem from doctors, social workers, or your relative's care coordinator: this is a common complaint.

In all these circumstances, you should try to remain calm. Becoming upset or angry will make things worse. It can be helpful to remember that your relative is not and was not always like this, and may not be aware of exactly how hurtful or upsetting their behaviour is. They may well be reacting in this way because they are actually very angry or frightened. Waiting until a particular outburst is over, and then saying 'I know you've been upset, what can I do to help?' has been found useful by others faced with this problem. It may be a good idea to leave the room, or to suggest that your relative goes to their own room or to another room just for a while. One son would often talk and swear to himself. The family managed to limit this by making it a rule that it should only happen in his bedroom.

It is often a good idea, after a particularly upsetting or embarrassing event, for the whole family, including your relative, to talk about it and work out ways of avoiding or limiting similar situations in the future. It is much better for all concerned if, when everyone is calm, you can make it clear to each other exactly what can be tolerated, and what will not be, rather than leaving things unsaid and letting irritation and upset build up.

Peter was in his early thirties, and sometimes when severely ill he would take his clothes off, regardless of who else was in the room. His mother and married sister, who lived with him, asked later why he did this and told him how upsetting it was for them. Peter said that sometimes he felt he was told to undress as an act of penitence, but agreed eventually to do it in private whenever possible. He needed reminding, but this worked reasonably well and was easier than coping with his behaviour or explaining it to visitors.

COPING WITH A DEPRESSED RELATIVE

If you live with someone who is mentally ill, maintaining the relationship while they are depressed can be one of the hardest things to manage. Depression saps the depressed person's will, and is quite capable of sapping yours too. It can be particularly exasperating to see your best efforts to help come to nothing, and it is not surprising that many relatives give up trying, and withdraw, emotionally at any rate. This unfortunately reinforces sufferers' sense of guilt and poor opinion of themselves, and emphasises how isolating depression can be.

However, although it may often be difficult, there are things you can do. The approach differs according to whether your relative is just becoming depressed, or whether the depression has really got a grip.

In the early stages of depression, it may be possible to improve things by using the sorts of approach that would be helpful for someone who was distressed or unhappy in the ordinary way. You may have to take the initiative though because depressed people may find it hard to confide. You can help by providing sympathy and sensible advice. For instance, if things at work are difficult, you may be able to see a way through the difficulties that your relative has missed, or persuade them to put them on one side until they are in a better position to deal with them. You may be able to provide practical support, reducing the load on your relative by taking on some task or responsibility on a temporary basis. One of the adverse effects of depression is to give people a distorted view of matters, which in turn makes the depression worse. By talking things through with them you may be able to provide them with a better perspective.

Reassurance is important to depressed people but it must not be done in a crude way. It is not reassuring for someone to have their fears and worries dismissed; it just makes them feel that the other person has not understood, or doesn't believe that their distress is real. It is much better to listen to the basis of the worries, to take them seriously, to spot where the sufferer is being unrealistic or oversensitive, and to put forward an alternative view. Your interest and concern will also help to reassure them of what they are very unsure of, that is, their worth.

When someone is depressed, people often feel they should try a change of scene. To this end they may suggest various social activities, or even a holiday. Unfortunately, this is often not a good idea, and in any case must be done very carefully. If it doesn't work and the person does not enjoy the occasion, it may bring home to them how impaired they are, and their depression may increase as a result. They may also feel guilty because they have spoilt things for others. Any social activity must therefore be planned in the light of the individual's state of mind. Simple visits by relatives or close friends may be all they can take and as much as they can benefit from at this stage

If your efforts to get your relative over their depression do not succeed in a week or two, you should enlist medical help, at first through your family doctor (GP), and if necessary you must press for psychiatric help. If your relative has had a depressive illness before, you may be quite a good judge of when things have gone too far, although it is often difficult to steer a course between tardiness and haste.

Even if your relative is getting assistance (for instance, someone to talk to and medication) from the professionals, there are still things you can do to help them. Indeed, it is important that you are not seen to give up in your attempts. Depressed people are rather unrewarding to be with, so there must always be a temptation for you to withdraw, and to a certain extent you may have to have time on your own just to keep going. As a result of their doubts about and poor opinion of themselves, some depressed people can be rather clinging and dependent, and this can also be difficult.

There comes a point when a depressed person cannot actually manage their responsibilities any more. When this has been reached, it is really up to you to take on these responsibilities yourself or organise others to do so. This means you must take charge and take over all household decisions without negotiation. Depressed people may be very indecisive. This may lead to long discussions about trivial matters that get nowhere because they continually change the basis of their argument. Such disputes are pointless, and you should avoid them or at least try and defer them. Sometimes sufferers become very opinionated about family matters, and this can also lead to long arguments that fail to produce constructive solutions.

Taking over like this may make your depressed relative feel very guilty at the burden they are placing on you. You can manage this by explaining that it is only a temporary arrangement, that when they are better, but not before, you will expect them to take things on once again, and that they would help you in the same way if you were in their circumstances. Depressed people often feel safer if they can feel that someone has taken firm control of the situation.

You need a certain skill to recognise the point at which you really have to take over. If you delay too long you may cause your relative a lot of unnecessary anguish. If you take over too early, you may be encouraging them to give up more than they have to.

In any case, even if you are doing most of the important things, you should still encourage your relative to do something, even though it does not seem worth the trouble it causes you.

Anne and her husband lived with her father Bob, who became depressed. Even though it was as much as he could manage she still got him to dry the dishes. He could only do this very slowly and under close supervision, but Anne still thought it was important that he should do it. It gave her something to thank him for, and it allowed him the feeling of a task done.

Another example of the use of simple activity to help someone who is depressed is given on page 127.

If your relative has become so depressed they cannot do anything at all, you must really consider whether they shouldn't be in hospital, or getting intensive home treatment. You certainly must not hide the situation from their doctor, and indeed you should make arrangements to discuss it with him or her.

In the vast majority of cases, depressed mood is temporary, so if you can last it out things will get better. Very occasionally depression may take the form of long lasting misery that seems unaffected by treatment. This is very difficult indeed to live with, and sometimes the only way to manage is to arrange matters in less than ideal ways. This might include taking over your relative's responsibilities, not on a temporary, but on a permanent basis. It also requires that you deliberately protect yourself from your relative's misery, at least for part of the time, by organising your life away from them to an extent. These courses of action will not do much to improve your relative's mood, but at least they may enable you to continue looking after them, and yourself.

COPING WITH DELUSIONS

One of the most difficult problems you might have to face occurs when your relative has a very firmly held belief: e.g. 'The television is talking to me". If you deny the truth of this belief, you may be seen to have joined 'them". If you agree with them, the belief can become even more fixed in the person's mind. You will find that arguing is not helpful. A useful strategy is for you to agree that your relative believes what he or she says, while making it clear that the experience is not real for you. 'I know you think the T.V. is talking to you, you are sensitive to that sort of thing at times. I don't find it talks to me", is one way of drawing a line between the person's own reality and the outside world.

Michael's wife could not at first understand what her husband meant when he said he was convinced that he had a special mission to fulfil. While agreeing with him and sympathising that he felt such urgency, she made it clear that it was not a belief she had, and that it was more important to her to have some help with a specific task (looking after their young son). This combination of sympathy (it is very important not to be dismissive) and distraction was successful some of the time in calming Michael and helping him not to act on his belief.

Sometimes, if you have a good relationship with your relative, reviewing the evidence for their belief with them can be helpful. This is not the same as trying to prove them wrong. It is not something to argue about. We do know however that once someone has a strong belief, be it about politics, religion, or world events, it is very common for them not to look closely at the evidence for another point of view. Particularly if your relative has a *distressing* belief, looking for disconfirming evidence together and reviewing it dispassionately can help to reassure them and reduce upset.

At times Peter thought that he was evil, and that if he were watching the news on T.V. he could cause the next disaster that was being reported. He often felt he knew what was going to be said next and that these thoughts then influenced world events, causing bad things to happen. Because he felt he was responsible for this, he often thought he should kill himself. His sister had tried to discuss these ideas with him but he was always totally convinced that his thoughts were the cause. However, one lunchtime, by discussing just beforehand what he thought was going to be on the news, they were both able to sit and watch it and see if his worst fears were confirmed or not. Peter said he knew that a terrible

Third World disaster was imminent, but in fact the news that day was about a political scandal. Suggesting to him that what he thought did not always happen helped to reassure him that he was not always to blame. It was not something Peter had been able to do for himself, but because his sister had discussed it with him beforehand, it helped relieve his distress. Peter began to see for himself that his worst forebodings did not inevitably come true and to reassure himself to some extent.

Discussing the evidence for a belief has to be done sympathetically and carefully or it can make your relative feel more convinced than ever. If you do try this sort of discussion, you must be able to leave off if it is clearly unhelpful or distressing, and try to reassure and distract your relative instead. 'It's all right, we don't have to talk about it if you don't want to' – and then change the subject. It may in the end be as helpful to switch off the news, or suggest another activity, if discussion is not possible with your relative at that moment.

RESTLESSNESS, OVERACTIVITY OR ANXIETY

Some people, particularly those with severe depression, can become extremely restless, uncomfortable and upset. They may be unable to sit still or to sleep, and spend hours pacing the room. No amount of reassurance seems to make any difference. You may well find this behaviour almost unbearable if it continues for long. It is nearly always helpful to acknowledge to your relative that they can't feel very comfortable or happy or relaxed either. Sometimes a walk outside together will be helpful; sometimes separate walks outside will be more so! Fortunately, symptoms of this type almost invariably get better as the illness recedes.

Pat, a mother of two in her forties, would sometimes feel unbearably anxious and upset, and ask constantly for reassurance that 'it was not her fault' and that she was not shouting obscenities. This was very difficult for her family to tolerate, as indeed it was for the staff when she went to hospital. Reassurance did no more than help her temporarily; indeed in the long run we know it can keep someone feeling anxious, as the relief of reassurance does not last. The feelings could last for days at a time. The best solution seemed to be to offer a brief stock phrase of reassurance, rather than to spend a long time trying to comfort her, and again to offer alternatives or distraction. Comments like 'we know how upset you are, try to sit down until you feel better' seemed to be helpful while this distressing behaviour was at its height. Trying to do things to reduce the anxiety itself, helping someone to relax and stay calm until the anxiety passes can be the most useful strategy.

EFFECTS ON SEXUAL RELATIONSHIPS

Those of you who are married to or cohabiting with someone who becomes severely mentally ill will be concerned about sexual aspects of the relationship. While they are unwell, many people, particularly those with severe depression, will lose much of their sexual desire and interest. Some types of drug treatment also tend to reduce sexual interest. This, together with a loss of more general expressions of affection, can be particularly difficult for partners to understand or accept. When the difficulties improve, sexual and general interest will probably return. You may however find that the relationship has been changed in sexual and other ways, and that new patterns must be established. You may also find that your feelings have changed irrevocably, and you may feel that the partnership cannot survive. Nearly all the partners we have talked to in this situation have wanted to end the relationship at one time or another, although the guilt this produces can be equally unbearable. Divorce is now common in our society, and for some relationships a severe mental illness is a final strain that cannot be tolerated. However some couples find that such experiences draw them closer together than they have been before.

Mary and her husband Bill were in their fifties but had not been married long. They found it very difficult at first to adjust when Bill developed a late onset type of schizophrenia. He had always had trouble staying in jobs, but this finally became much worse after a particularly damaging row with his boss, following which he refused to leave the house and was very disturbed. Eventually, after treatment in hospital, he returned home, and they had to decide how their relationship ought to continue. Mary's first impulse was to give up her career to 'look after Bill'. Bill did not want her to do this, and felt she would resent it in the long run. Eventually they decided that Mary should continue working part-time while Bill began to take on some of the domestic responsibilities instead of trying and failing at jobs. Bill's new role took some time to establish, but he began to enjoy it and gained a sense of achievement from having dinner ready for a tired wife. Mary was actually very glad to relinquish the housework, and also to have time to spend with him on days she was not at work. They both finally described the relationship as very close, and as more fulfilling, including sexually, in the way it had developed.

PROMISCUITY

Particularly if you are a parent, you may be worried by the fact that promiscuous behaviour may become a problem. A much loved child, who may have been shy before the illness began, seems to lose discrimination and chooses as sexual partners people who would previously have been considered as unlikely or unsuitable in some way. Sometimes you will feel particularly concerned because your son or daughter appears vulnerable to sexual advances, and you might worry that outsiders could be taking advantage. This can be a very upsetting problem: you find that your normal acceptance of an adult's desire for independence and sexual freedom conflicts with your need to protect a loved child from sexual abuse or hurt. For adults with mental illness, there is rarely any way to enforce sexual rules. Even though you dislike it, you may have to accept a certain amount of independence and sexual freedom. The most useful approach is to support your relative through these relationships, showing you still care, despite their acting in ways you would not choose them to. Help with safe sex and contraception is usually relevant and important, and you may be the person best able to suggest and organise this.

Most families, particularly parents, find it very difficult to accept this side of their relatives' adult life.

The parents of Mary, a woman in her early thirties, were distressed by her going off for several nights with an unknown man, after which she had returned home dishevelled and uncommunicative. They never did hear the full details of this episode. Thereafter they tended to be rather protective of her, and discouraged male friends from phoning or calling round.

In this family Mary herself was not worried by her lack of a boyfriend, and she did not disagree with her parents' attitude. It can be much more difficult if this becomes an area of dispute in your family, because it has to be sorted out in some way that respects your relative's adult needs.

In some cases, promiscuity may only be apparent for some of the time. This can happen in mania, where it might be an early sign of relapse, and you may need to enlist urgent professional help. We give advice on how to do this on page .

DIET

There is no good evidence that dietary factors can cause schizophrenia or bipolar disorder. We are all bombarded with new facts about food and diets, but very little seems to relate to mental health specifically. Psychiatric disorders can result from deficiencies of vitamins, but these are quite different and, in addition, can often be recognised by their effects on your relative's physical health. However, many people with severe mental illness do have a poor diet, and it is important for their relatives to ensure as far as possible that they have a sensible diet, containing a range of food and including the essential nutrients.

Some people with mental health problems eat too much, and, as they may also be rather underactive, this can lead to obesity. More worryingly, it has become clear recently that individuals taking major tranquillisers, antidepressants, or lithium may be liable to put on weight; with some medication this can be up to 8 kilos in a year. As with anyone else, it is not sensible to get too fat. You should try and encourage your relative to lose weight, although this may be quite difficult in some cases, and may appear to be the least of their problems. Sometimes the doctor may be able to change your relative to drugs that are less fattening, and it can be helpful to ask about this, if you think it is a problem.

SELF-CARE

This is not a problem for everyone with mental health problems. However, for some people, there is a loss of interest in how they look, and how they look after themselves. In extreme cases, self-neglect may be severe, with the person not eating properly and living in squalor. This is, however, not usually allowed to happen if they live with a relative! Nevertheless, there are often day to day problems over bathing or shaving, and there may be a difficulty about changing clothes, particularly underwear. One mother described how her son became attached to particular set of clothes he had on and would not change them. All she could do was to persuade him to bathe about once a month, and to wash these clothes while he was doing so. When eventually they wore out, the same thing happened to the new set. It is helpful in these circumstances to establish family ground rules for a minimum routine of bathing, laundering, changing of sheets, that you can all at any rate tolerate. Once a week may be a reasonable target, and, once negotiated, your relative can be encouraged to stick to it. It can be useful to decide on a particular convenient day and include bathing as part of a general routine of getting up, getting dressed and getting out of the house. It may well need your practical help to start off with, as shaving or hair washing may be particularly burdensome for someone feeling very pre-occupied or upset.

USE OF ALCOHOL

While there is no intrinsic reason why someone who has had a severe mental illness cannot drink alcohol, it may be inadvisable for several reasons. First, anyone taking drugs such as the major tranquillisers needs to be aware they interact with alcohol. This can cause an exaggeration of the normal effects of alcohol, and the individual may quickly become sleepy, morose, or less in control of strong emotions such as anger or fear.

Even doctors normally recommend that anyone on psychiatric drugs should drink very little alcohol, if indeed any. However, this may be quite unrealistic. Your relative may greatly resent being given 'rules' about drinking, whether by professionals or even by you. They may rightly feel that alcohol is one of the few pleasures they now enjoy. In general, a couple of pints of beer or two or three glasses of wine every other day should not cause too many problems. As a rule of thumb, your relative should try to think of their drugs as doubling the potency of alcohol, so the effect of a pint of beer is likely to equal that of two pints in former times. It may be that a little cautious experimentation is required. As with the rest of us, some people with mental health problems have much more control over their alcohol consumption than others. Calm discussion about the problems excessive use of alcohol can cause them and the other members of the family is probably the best starting point. If alcohol is causing serious problems, the GP or team concerned with your relative's care should be told about it, in case they have minimised or denied the difficulties.

Some families, fortunately not a majority, find that worrying about a relative's alcohol consumption and their resulting behaviour can be one of the worst aspects they have to deal with. Your relative may well not drink to what would normally be regarded as excess, but because even small amounts of alcohol can have effects when combined with medication, the results of quite moderate drinking can be very unpleasant. John lived with his mother, and would nag and worry her every night for money for a few beers. He would consume these and then return home drunk and be sick over the bed. It took a lot of negotiation between John, his mother and the mental health team before this pattern was changed, and he could behave in a more acceptable manner.

A different strategy was developed by Eric's mother. When Eric said he wanted a bottle of whisky, his mother would suggest that they both needed a drink and offer to buy one on her next shopping trip. She would do this, and for a few nights afterwards, they had a couple of drinks together. After that Eric lost interest, and the bottle remained half full in the cupboard.

SUBSTANCE ABUSE

As well as alcohol, taking street drugs is part of the leisure activities of increasing numbers of people, particularly in their teens and twenties. Cannabis, 'E', amphetamines, and LSD may be used, as indeed may heroin, cocaine or 'crack'. While there is some argument about causes and effects, heavy consumption of these drugs, with the possible exception of heroin, almost certainly increase the risk of psychosis. There is now strong evidence that cannabis, particularly if consumed heavily in the teenage years, makes an onset of psychosis up to three times more likely, with most impact on those with a family history of psychosis. At the very least all substance abuse exaggerates the problems of someone with psychosis, and often seem to set off another episode. People who become dependent on a particular illicit drug, such as heroin or amphetamines, may find that they also acquire all the associated difficulties, such as having to find the money needed to get the drugs, and becoming less and less concerned with anything else while they search for the next fix.

Recent research on people with psychosis who are also heavy users of street drugs or alcohol indicates they have even more frequent emergencies and problems. Such substance abuse is likely to need help in its own right, separately from the problems caused by schizophrenia or severe depression. Because of this, you may well need to be aware of the possibility of this happening to your relative and be ready to contact your GP for specialist advice on the drug or alcohol problem. Unfortunately, as with all addictions, the only way to help someone is to lead them to recognise that they themselves need to change, and this may take many years of disaster and heartache. Such combined problems are some of the most difficult to deal with. If you are in this position, try to obtain all the help you can, both for your relative and yourself. However, you may also need to recognise that there are limits to what you can do. You may only be able to provide a 'safety net' until your relative decides for themselves to seek some help.

THREATS OF SUICIDE

Schizophrenia and manic depressive illness are both associated with a higher than average risk of attempted or actual suicide. Sometimes suicidal feelings may be a near-rational response to hopeless circumstances, but in other cases there may be no apparent cause. One of the reasons that the mental health team may suggest intensive home treatment or a hospital admission is to reduce the risk of suicide and help such feelings recede. Sometimes people are most at risk of attempting suicide when there has been some initial improvement. They may feel a bit more energetic, but still believe that they are a burden to others, that they have nothing to live for and that the future is completely bleak. It is not possible to prevent all suicide attempts: a determined individual can often be successful, even when under apparently close surveillance in a home, a hostel or a hospital ward.

Fred, a depressed middle aged man, was being monitored in hospital because he was regarded as a suicide risk. He wanted to use the toilet, but while he was there, the nurse watching him was called briefly to a disturbance on the ward. Although he was only gone a moment, when he returned Fred had thrown himself out of the small toilet window, three floors up.

Threats of suicide can be very upsetting and difficult to deal with. It is commonly said that people who talk frequently about suicide never actually try to kill themselves. This is not true: *all threats of suicide should be taken seriously*. It is true that people sometimes make such threats for effect or because it is the only way they can communicate how distressed they are. At other times, they most certainly are seriously intent on killing themselves, and you may find it impossible to tell one kind of threat from another. It is sensible to take elementary precautions, such as not leaving tablets lying around the house and informing the GP or mental health team if your relative seems more than normally tearful, morose or hopeless. You may find it helpful to ask them how they are feeling, as sometimes it is just necessary to notice the sadness and attempt to offer comfort and reassurance, if it will be accepted. An arm round the shoulders or a cuddle may sometimes be easier than words, and often more effective.

DEALING WITH AND ANTICIPATING EMERGENCIES

It is in the nature of severe mental illness that you may sometimes be called upon to deal with urgent situations. The appropriate management of these depends on the exact circumstances.

Probably the most common situation is when you become aware that your relative is relapsing; their mental health is rapidly deteriorating. It is always possible and often appropriate to seek the advice of your family doctor (the GP) about this. You may be able to persuade your relative to make an appointment. It will be helpful if you can accompany them. Sometimes, they may decline to see your family doctor. This may be because they have particular fears about what may happen, for instance that they will have to go into hospital, perhaps never to come out, or that they will be sectioned and taken to hospital involuntarily. If they are reluctant, it is worth trying to find out what they feel about going to see the GP – you may be able to reassure them and get them to change their mind, particularly if you offer to go with them. If you are completely unable to get them to visit the surgery, it is reasonable for you to make an appointment and see the GP yourself. If you decide that this is necessary, there is plainly no point in doing it half-heartedly – you must put your doctor clearly in the picture. Otherwise, he or she may feel that you have just come for some reassurance. The GP may make a home visit if it seems reasonable to do so from what you tell them.

If your relative is currently attending a psychiatric outpatient department, the best procedure may be to consult the psychiatrist involved by phone. The psychiatrist may sometimes be in a position to reassure you. However, if a genuine crisis is developing, they can suggest the best course of action, whether this is a temporary increase in medication, or even more intensive home treatment or a hospital admission. Your relative may be receiving visits from a Community Psychiatric Nurse, or whichever member of the mental health team is their care coordinator (see Ch. 3). They will nearly always know them better than the psychiatrist. In these circumstances, it is sensible to contact the care coordinator who may decide to make an urgent visit to assess the situation. Care coordinators should routinely provide instructions about how best to contact them, and you should ensure you know how to do this before a crisis arises. In cases of doubt, the consultant psychiatrist's secretary will usually know how to get a message to them. It is worth having these numbers by the phone or in your mobile phone as a precaution.

In some circumstances you may feel it is sufficient for your relative's next appointment to be brought forward. This can usually be done, either through the appointments secretary at the hospital, or by phoning the relevant community mental health team, who will have a duty worker who can always take a message or arrange an appointment directly.

Not all service users need to remain permanently in contact with mental health services. It is usually appropriate for relatives of those showing signs of relapse or deterioration after a long period of good health to approach their family doctor. Services are now organised through GPs, who are linked to health service organisations called Primary Care Trusts. Family doctors prefer patients to visit them in their surgery, as this is usually the most effective way for them to use their time. However, for some service users this may be inappropriate, so it may sometimes be in order to ask your GP to visit your relative at home. Sometimes, after seeing them, the GP may decide to arrange intensive home treatment, crisis treatment or a hospital admission immediately. Otherwise, an out-patient appointment to see a consultant in the new team may be arranged. If your relative is unwilling or unable to attend, or needs to be seen quickly, your family doctor may invite a consultant to visit them in the home (a domiciliary visit).

If you have moved house you may need to change GP; if so, it is important to do this quickly. Moving may mean that the mental health services (secondary services) responsible for your relative also change. If your relative is currently in contact with mental health services, someone from the service will usually organise a transfer of care to a new service serving the area you are moving to. Otherwise, contacting your relative's new GP is usually the first step.

Occasionally, your relative may become very acutely disturbed. Where there are warning signs of this, it is obviously better to take action early rather than late. Sometimes, however, people deteriorate very rapidly and you may need to do something immediately. If you have a particularly good relationship with the hospital or mental health consultant, admission to hospital can sometimes be put in motion by contacting him or her directly. Otherwise, it may be necessary to obtain the services of your GP who can assess the situation in the home and arrange a necessary admission accordingly. Sometimes, these relatively urgent situations arise when you and your relative are away from home. Under these circumstances, you may need to enlist the help of a local, temporary, GP, who in turn may arrange admission to a nearby hospital to start with. Your relative can then be transferred to their own local services when it is convenient and practicable.

In a few areas there are Special Crisis Intervention Centres or Emergency Clinics, where you can go to get help without necessarily contacting your family doctor. Many general hospitals now run a liaison service with psychiatry, and so attending your local Accident & Emergency Department may mean your relative will be assessed. However, although the government has managed to reduce waiting times, there will still often be something of a long wait. If at all possible, find out beforehand from your community mental health team what you should do in an out-of-hours emergency, and try to keep the relevant contact numbers easily available. If you are seriously worried about your safety or that of your relative and it is an emergency, you will need to phone 999 and ask for the police. Many relatives have told us this is the most reliable way to get help late at night.

Sometimes people are so disturbed they deny that they have become unwell. In these circumstances, they may need compulsory admission to prevent them from harming themselves or other people. This should be arranged through the community mental health team, a special crisis intervention team or the family doctor. Some details of the legal involvement of the relative in the procedures of compulsory admission are given in Chapter Six.

If your relative is very disturbed and leaves the house, and you are seriously worried, it is reasonable to inform the local police. They can act under the 1983 Mental Health Act or the Scottish or Northern Irish equivalents to bring a person suffering from a mental illness who is likely to be a danger to themselves or others to a 'place of safety' (see page 146).

The final emergency you may have to face arises from an attempt at suicide by your relative.

Most such attempts these days involve self-poisoning. Not all are equally serious but you should seek medical help if there is *any possibility* at all that your relative could have swallowed more than a usual dose of a drug, or that they retain an intention to end their life. Some drugs like paracetamol (Panadol) can be fatal in overdose after a delay, even though they appear to have no immediate effects. In the case of any overdose, you should seek general medical, rather than psychiatric, help. Family doctors usually do not have adequate facilities for dealing with overdosage, although they can help to assess the severity of the overdose and advise whether the patient needs to be taken to hospital. If there is any suspicion that the overdose might be a dangerous one, you should either take your relative to an Accident & Emergency Department at your local hospital or phone 999 for an ambulance.

COPING WITH VIOLENT BEHAVIOUR

We live in what is perhaps an increasingly violent society, but relatively few mentally ill people are in any way violent. It must be said however that the ones who are do get a lot of publicity. Nevertheless, violence in the mentally ill does pose some rather special problems for the people who live with them. As with all violence, it is more likely to be directed at someone already known to your relative than a stranger. Especially if you live with them it is worth thinking this through and trying to prevent violence from occurring or escalating.

The next thing to be acknowledged about violence, however, is that, like suicide, it is not always preventable. There are sometimes going to be situations where it erupts without anyone being able to do anything to stop it. In the worst possible case, a pattern of repeated violence may be so established, for instance between a powerful adult son and his ageing frail mother, that it is not possible to change it. In such cases, it may be necessary to stop living together, and even for you to take such actions as changing the locks or getting a court injunction against your relative.

However, things are not usually as bad as that, and action can be taken to deal with the violent behaviour. This action has three aspects, depending on whether it is to do with anticipating the violence, deals with the act itself, or takes place in the aftermath.

Effective action taken before someone actually behaves aggressively is obviously to be preferred. If you know that your relative is particularly irritable and therefore in a mood that may lead to violence, you may be able to avoid triggering it. One way of doing this is simple avoidance – keep out of their way, go to another room, go out for a walk or to the cinema. Sometimes, you may have noticed that certain topics or situations tend to make your relative angry: obviously these should be avoided if possible. The strategy of avoidance can be quite effective, but it may have the drawback that nothing in the situation is changed, especially as it is not usually possible to keep the avoidance up for ever. One relative had learnt to recognise when tension was building up in her son from the expression on his face. When this happened, she would keep quiet and leave the room. However, it was obviously not always possible for her to stay out of the living room.

A somewhat more subtle policy is of deflection: if tension seems to be building up in your relative it may be possible to defuse it by suggesting some simple routine activity, going to the shops or doing some household chore. This obviously requires sensitivity and good judgement, as the wrong choice may make the situation worse. Some-times, relatives learn by experience that certain phrases are calming, and can be used to defuse the situation. One family would say 'why don't you go and have a lie down'. Sometimes this would work, but at other times, the suggestion would be received angrily. It then worked better to say 'well go out and buy *me* some cigarettes/newspaper – here's the money – and come back when you feel calmer'.

A more direct approach is to confront your relative with their anger: this must be done very gently. One way of doing it is by saying in a quiet and neutral tone something like, 'I can see you are upset. Won't you tell me what's the matter?' This may sound trite, but at least it gives your relative the chance of talking about their angry feelings, rather than necessarily acting on them. Again, this requires very fine judgement, but it also carries the possibility of sorting the situation out in a more basic and complete way.

Sometimes your relative may become violent because they have misinterpreted things. This may be the sort of misinterpretation that any of us can make, but which those who are upset and distressed may make more easily, or it can be the result of delusional ideas. In either case, if you realise that your relative is becoming angry because of misinterpretation, you may be able to clarify the situation by gentle questioning. If the misinterpretation is not a delusional one, it may be possible for you to clear things up. If it is delusional, it may help to draw lines between your relative's reality and your own, or to look at the evidence together, in the manner suggested on page 45. However far you can get with clarifying misinterpretations, it is important to keep the transaction quiet and calm, using a firm and unflustered voice. If you can give the impression that you aren't going to become upset or angry, this will give your relative the feeling that things are under control, and this in turn will exert a calming influence. On some days one daughter would keep bursting in to her mother shouting threateningly: 'I know you're trying to kill me. Why are you making me feel ill?' Her mother had learnt that one response that would calm her down was to say firmly but clearly: 'No I was just sitting here reading the paper. Please don't shout'. It was often helpful to use distraction as well. 'Why don't we go out for a walk/make a cup of tea?'

Very often violence is a response to frustration – it arises when you feel you must refuse something your relative wants. This may happen sometimes anyway, but it is more likely if the ground rules of your relationship have not been made very clear. So, for example, if you appear to have been inconsistent about what you think is all right and what not, violence may be the method your relative uses to get you to permit what you would really rather like to refuse. This underlines the importance of firmness and clarity in your relationship. Your relative may be quite disturbed, but they will still be able to recognise this firmness and realise that there are limits beyond which they cannot pass. Knowing where they stand in this way may actually help them feel safer. Firmness in this sense is not to be confused with bossiness or intrusiveness. 'We agreed how much money you should have each day. I can't give you any more', said with conviction, confidently and consistently when the previously agreed limit has been reached is one example of the right sort of firmness.

However, consistency may be an ideal, but it is not all that easy to achieve, particularly if the situation has been going on for a long time and you have not been able to get help and guidance. If you have been inconsistent in the past, sadly, the pattern may be impossible to modify. Inconsistency in one relative going hand in hand with violence in the other is a frequent cause of family break-up, although the relationship may stagger painfully on for a long time before this eventually happens. Usually when there is a break-up, the carer feels extremely guilty, even though the decision was the only realistic and practicable one to take. The relationship in our experience which most frequently gets locked into violence in this way is that between a mother, often elderly, and her ill but vigorous son: however, it can happen in most types of relationship, and we also know of caring husbands who have been intimidated by their wives' violence.

You may be quite skilful at managing your relationship with your mentally ill relative, and yet there are still times when they become violent with you. It is just not possible to be completely in control of the situation all the time. After all, professional staff are hit and hurt by service users from time to time, and it can become a question of just being in the wrong place at the wrong time.

So how can you deal with the immediate threat or the fact of violence? It helps if you have thought out beforehand what you will do, and what you are prepared to do. It obviously depends to a major extent on how able you are to withstand an assault physically. The first principle is that immediately you become aware that you might be about to be attacked, you should avoid getting stuck in the corner of the room. Try and keep the furniture between you and your relative. Leave the room if necessary and if possible. If you can't get out, as a last resort use a chair or a blanket or jacket as a defence. You may need to leave the house and call or phone for help. It may help to have made an arrangement with a neighbour beforehand. Do not be afraid to call the police if necessary.

Unfortunately, people like social workers or the police may not be able to do very much before violence has actually occurred. This may seem crazy, but is of course the other side of our civil liberties in this country.

However, the police will often at least appear on the scene, and having several police officers around will frequently calm things down, even to the extent that when they have to leave your relative does not become so angry again. This matter of calling the police does require judgement – if you get to the stage where your relative is continually having outbursts of rage and violence and you are continually calling in the police, this is no proper basis for your relationship. You must get outside advice urgently, preferably from a mental health professional involved in your relative's care, and if the circumstances cannot be changed for the better, you must seriously consider parting company.

Sometimes there may be no escape or possibility of help, and the threat of violence may be so immediate and dangerous that you have to comply with doing things you don't want to. This is particularly the case if your relative has a knife or a gun, but also applies if they are much bigger and stronger than you.

If your relative has actually been violent towards you, hit you or whatever, it is important to try and deal with it afterwards in a way that may reduce its recurrence. It is relatively unusual to be badly hurt, but it obviously can happen. Being hit is, however, often very upsetting even when the physical damage is slight, because it says something to you about your relationship, and also about the future – that it may be unpleasant, violent, and uncontrollable.

It is important that you should gently but firmly confront your relative with the fact that they have been violent and upset you. You should do this later, when they have had time to settle down – perhaps the next day. Most acts of violence occur in the evening or at night time, and talking about it during daylight has a normalising effect. You should point out that you were hurt and upset by their behaviour – they may not realise the effect it has had on you. You should then try to get them to apologise – this emphasises to them that they have gone beyond acceptable limits. At the same time you should explore the incident and try to find out why it happened. Your relative may have been angry as a response to being very frightened, and your reassurance may be very helpful. They may also have felt that you were being unreasonable in some way. You may be able to explain the situation and your view of it to them in a way that is reassuring. It may then be possible to resolve your differences. Your relative may also have been triggered into violence by alcohol, substance abuse, or even lack of sleep. Pinpointing particular triggers can help avoid future episodes.

Finally, acts of violence often mean that your relative is relapsing, and this may require you to take further action (see page 53).

MONEY PROBLEMS

Some people with severe mental illness become very unrealistic about money. This is particularly true of the manic phases of bipolar disorder, and some of you may know that problems are returning because your relative draws out large amounts of money from an account and goes on a spending spree. Other people may not be able to get a job, and rely totally on social security or sickness benefit. They may find it impossible to budget, and demand extra money from you to pay for cigarettes, illicit drugs, alcohol or daily necessities. You may find these demands difficult to refuse, but resent the fact your relative cannot be more responsible or independent. Sometimes a daily budget can be organised with them, so that money is spaced out over the week and not spent all at once. Jane was able to agree with her mother that she should have £5 a day for herself. Clothing and other items were bought rarely, but out of their joint money. Gradually, as Jane became better at managing, it was possible to phase out this daily allowance system.

Partners may find money problems particularly worrying. If the illness prevents one or both of you from working, financial problems can indeed cause great hardship, particularly if there are young children. Sometimes it will be realistic for partners to change roles, so the person with mental ill health helps in the home while the other partner goes out to work. Often even simple household tasks will be too much for your relative, especially just after returning home from hospital, and other friends and carers may have to help with child care and housework.

People sometimes fail to claim all the benefits to which they are entitled, and your relative may need your help in such matters. Some guidance is given on this at the end of this chapter.

WHAT CAN BE DONE IF YOUR RELATIVE CANNOT MANAGE THEIR AFFAIRS BECAUSE OF MENTAL ILLNESS?

If you are worried because your relative seems to be getting into difficulties in managing money or property, you may suggest to them that they take out a Power of Attorney authorizing you or another person to handle their property. This is a legal document which your solicitor will help you with. It depends on your relative being able to understand what is meant by signing the document, and if they become mentally capable afterwards, the power is revoked. They may also revoke it themselves at any time. If your relative is so mentally disordered that their power of attorney would be invalid, you can apply to the *Court of Protection*. This is part of the Supreme Court and is staffed by judges. The website is given in the appendix, and the Court itself will advise you about the correct procedure. It will assess the medical evidence and may appoint a *Receiver*. The Receiver may be a court official but is usually a relative or close friend. They have control over the patient's property, and duties such as investing money, settling debts and keeping property in good repair. The Court can also conduct legal business for the patient, such as divorce proceedings or making a will. Unlike an ordinary Power of Attorney, the patient cannot revoke this arrangement. Patients must be told of an application to the Court of Protection, and can object if they think it is unreasonable. They must then write to the Court within seven days of being informed or before the hearing, whichever is the later. They may provide their own medical witnesses to their fitness.

The Court of Protection does have a duty to be cautious. In our experience, this can sometimes make it a rather inflexible and bureaucratic organisation. For this reason, it is best to invoke its help only when it has become absolutely necessary, as it may later make decisions that you cannot change and would not have wished.

CHILDREN IN THE FAMILY

A recent report (NSPCC, 2002) found that up to half of those with mental health problems may be parents. You may worry that children will be adversely affected by the strain of living with someone suffering a severe mental illness. It is, of course, impossible to rule this out, particularly if problems lead to financial or other hardships, or to upsets like having to move house or change schools frequently. However, many children have to cope with these things regardless of their parent's mental health. Getting help from neighbours, friends and other relatives may be crucial in relieving strains, and will mean that children have other adults to turn to if required. This can be particularly important. Some reasonable and simple explanation should always be given even to younger children. Confusing messages about 'daddy or mummy going away' without any reason being given can make children feel insecure and upset, or even that in some way it is their fault. It may be helpful to talk to children in a period of calm about some of the experiences that the parent had. The experiences can be compared to being in a dream, not necessarily a pleasant one, that continues even when the parent is awake. This can be used to explain why they may be preoccupied or upset, or seem less caring or interested in the child. Older children can themselves often be supportive, if they are given a chance to understand the problems, and if difficulties are dealt with calmly so that upsetting or frightening crises can be avoided. If problems do become too difficult, families with dependent children will normally be given prompt help from professionals, such as the local children's social services department, child guidance clinic, or the community mental health team if your relative is a service user. More recently, self help groups for child carers have been set up for a range of conditions, including severe mental health problems. Your local mental health team, or RETHINK may know of any local resources available (see appendices).

Occasionally problems in the family where there are children may seem insurmountable. Social services are now part of local mental health teams. In these circumstances, the community mental health team will contact the child protection team and they will be called in to assess the situation. Their aim is always to focus on the wellbeing of the child. This usually means that they will try to support a child within their family home. They may be able to offer domestic help or a substitute carer who lives in while a parent is in hospital, or while a parent is at work. In exceptional circumstances children may be temporarily received into the care of the local authority and placed with foster parents or in a children's home. This would only occur if there was no familiar alternative person, such as another relative or friend, who was able and suitable to care for them. Social services can also pay for temporary carers if there are financial difficulties.

Another worry that affects families is the possibility that children may inherit a tendency for the disorder. This risk is real, but differs according to the exact circumstances. The worst situation is very unusual, and is when both parents have a severe mental illness. In this case, around half of their children will be affected. Normally, only one parent has a severe mental illness. Overall, the risk that a child with one parent affected and one unaffected by, say, schizophrenia, will themselves develop the illness is about 10%, but this varies. The risk is less when schizophrenia in the parent is associated with a recognisable non-inherited cause, like birth injury, or, later on, head injury or epilepsy. It is also less if there is no-one else in the family with these problems. The risk is greater when the parent's schizophrenia is of a severe type.

Bipolar disorder also runs in families. For bipolar and severe unipolar illnesses this is mainly because it is inherited, not because people in families tend to share troubles and difficulties that might cause depression. The inherited risk for bipolar disorder is probably about the same as for schizophrenia, that for unipolar disorder somewhat less.

The fact that these disorders are partly inherited can raise the question of whether people who develop them should choose to have children if they haven't already done so. Most professionals would feel that the genetic risk in the majority of cases is of a degree that should not necessarily deter possible parents. Obviously this is a decision that must be taken by the couple, and the genetic risk is only one consideration. More important is whether the problems seriously undermine the person's ability to carry out the duties and everyday responsibilities of parenthood.

Finally, there is no reason why unaffected brothers and sisters of a person with one of these conditions should not themselves have children: here the genetic risk is very small indeed.

In some centres, it is possible to get advice on these matters from a special Genetic Counselling Service. It may be worth asking if there is one in your area.

RELAPSE

In most cases, particularly if relapse (a recurrence of the illness) has occurred before, you will be the best judge of whether your problems are recurring. However, some pointers may be useful, as these difficulties may reappear, and sometimes the development of the relapse may not closely resemble the original way the problem presented itself.

Relapses are recognised by changes in behaviour. One of the problems in spotting the early stages of relapse is that changes often happen gradually. This means that it may be very difficult to distinguish between normal behaviour and that due to the difficulties recurring.

For example, one of the changes that occur in mania is increased irritability. If someone loses their temper, it is often hard to tell if this is a normal response, or a bit excessive for that person in these particular circumstances. This is the sort of judgement you are liable to be extremely good at, given that you live with the person all the time. Indeed one of the common complaints levelled at clinical staff is that they do not believe that relatives can pick up such subtle changes, and so do not act upon the information, thus failing to prevent a crisis from developing.

What symptoms should you look out for? In schizophrenia, small changes in someone's normal pattern can give a clue. The person may stay up into the small hours of the morning, sometimes compensating by getting up later. They may go off their food, or eat in a more faddy way. They may spend increasing amounts of time on their own, shying away from the company of the family or of visitors. They may not look after themselves so well and behave in awkward or obstinate ways. They may be increasingly suspicious and wary. They may smile less and become more distant. A chance remark may suggest that they are returning to the preoccupations they had when they were unwell. One wife knew that her husband was relapsing when he lost interest in going to the day centre, spent more and more time in bed, and began talking again of 'the spies' on the TV programmes. In many people with schizophrenia, relapse is heralded by the sorts of feelings of tenseness and nervousness that we all experience from time to time, but which in them may mean something more worrying.

The major changes may be of mood: they may be increasingly nervous or depressed. However, people with schizophrenia sometimes become depressed without it indicating relapse: they may well have enough to be depressed about, so it can be hard to distinguish these reactions to an unrewarding situation from the symptoms of relapse.

Relapse in unipolar depression is often gradual. The person slowly becomes less energetic, doing less about the house. They lose pleasure in things that usually please them. They become quieter and less sociable. They may have trouble getting off to sleep or wake much too early in the morning. They take less pleasure in eating and may eat less, leaving food on the plate. They may surprise you by bursting into tears in response to what seemed a fairly harmless remark.

In contrast, the return of mania may be suggested by an increased energy. The person becomes noticeably more jovial, and may start to make plans or organise things. One woman's husband knew she was relapsing when she took over the task of walking the dog and began to make slightly unrealistic plans for a return to full-time work. Alteration in sleep patterns are often a clear early sign – typically people suddenly need less sleep. Your relative may begin to stay up late and be more talkative than usual. They may eat more and hurry their food. They may also become more irritable. They may go without sleep for one or two nights. This latter is often a clear warning sign.

If you think your relative is relapsing, you must try to take action. Some guidance is given on page 53.

All the changes described above can be seen in a fully fledged relapse. In the early stages, they are much less pronounced. This makes a real problem for you. On one hand, if you can recognise a relapse early, it can be nipped in the bud by prompt treatment. On the other, it makes a relationship difficult if you are always on the alert for signs of relapse and everything your relative does is evaluated to see if it is normal or not. Obviously a balance has to be struck, and you will have to reach this in the light of your own particular experiences. Some services try to discuss early worrying signs of a relapse as part of the care programme approach, and you may be able to ensure that a phone call from you is included as part of this pattern. (We will discuss this process later page 68.) You may also be able to discuss this calmly with your relative: What would you like to happen if things get worse again? What should I do? What would you want? These can all be helpful questions.

If your relative starts refusing to take their medication, a relapse may become more likely over the next few months. This is a problem looked at in more detail under treatments in chapter four.

GETTING AROUND THE BENEFITS SYSTEM.

We originally had a detailed section given over to this topic, but we have not included it in this edition, as terminology and benefits change constantly and quickly get out of date. You can find up-to-date help at your Citizens Advice Bureau (local 'phone book) and the local mental health team may well have a benefits advisor who will be a specialist in this area. If you are having problems do contact your relative's care coordinator to ask for help. If you do not have contact with a local team ask RETHINK or Mind (see appendix) for advice.

The Benefits and Work website provides free guides about all aspects of available benefits, including disability living allowance, attendance allowance, and incapacity benefit. The website is for people with long-term physical or mental health conditions, but also for carers.

3   Community Care

The development of community care started around fifty years ago. In fact, the number of inpatients in mental hospitals in the UK peaked in 1954. This meant there were increasing numbers of people living in the community who previously were, or would have been, in mental hospitals. Some of these people were able to live at home because of innovative programmes of rehabilitation and accommodation. However, in many cases, it just meant placing additional burdens on carers. The process of reducing hospital beds accelerated in the 1980s. However, the services developed at that time to deal with the community care for people with severe mental illness always lagged behind what was needed. Services were very rarely linked together so that they could work efficiently for the benefit of clients.

The Care Programme Approach (CPA) was introduced in 1991 to provide a framework for the care of mentally ill people outside hospitals. Since then, health and social services have merged into local mental health teams. These are now the basis for setting up arrangements for the care and treatment of people with severe mental health problems in the community. The Care Programme Approach (CPA) requires that services provide a needs assessment which in turn leads to a care plan, agreed with the service user, and which covers needs over the next 6 months to a year. This has to be put into practice and reviewed regularly. The person responsible for coordinating this is called a care coordinator. This person might be a social worker, a community psychiatric nurse (CPN) or occasionally an occupational therapist (OT) (see Chapter 4). The care coordinator is required to keep in close touch with the service user and to make sure that the programme is going well. Care coordinators have a large number of responsibilities. They have to organise all aspects of care, even though they may not carry them out themselves. They have to form the main therapeutic relationship with their clients and try to ensure that they both receive and accept the treatment they need. They act as a channel of communication between the client and the community mental health team. They also liaise with outside agencies, such as housing or benefit offices. These days they are required to keep in touch with service users even if they go into prison. If service users are on an enhanced level of the CPA, they are required to have a care coordinator even if they move, or are difficult to get hold of. Care coordinators are required to try to maintain some sort of contact with them, or arrange their transfer to a new area, until they are discharged from the care programme. Finally, they act as advocate, advisor and friend to their clients.

Another thing that the Care Programme Approach has done is to formalise the idea of team working. Multidisciplinary teams have existed here and there for at least twenty years. They have been an effective way of using the various sorts of knowledge and expertise of different professional groups: community psychiatric nurses, doctors, clinical psychologists, occupational therapists, and social workers.

The Care Programme Approach (CPA) in theory gives very powerful official recognition to the involvement of carers in a major way in planning treatment and services for their relatives. The CPA guidelines say that carers' contributions to meeting client's needs should be explicitly recognised in the care plan. The National Service Framework for Mental Health, published in 1999, says that people providing regular and substantial care for someone on the CPA should have an assessment of their own caring, physical and mental health needs, repeated on at least an annual basis. They should have their own written care plan, which is to be given to them and implemented in discussion with them. The Carer and Disabled Children Act 2000, which came into force in 2001, gives all non-professional carers (ie. not only the carers of people with mental health problems) the right to an assessment of their needs. It requires local authorities to provide services and care that supports them in their caring role and monitors their health and well being. This help should include meeting carers' needs for support, periods of respite care, and 24-hour access to an emergency mental health service.

It must be said that, so far, these represent aspirations rather than realities. This has led to some frustration. Recent criticisms of carer assessments suggest that they are often felt to be token, and are not matched by resources. However, the main purpose of assessments was always to ensure that local teams became more aware of carers and had discussions with them. They were thus to become a 'driving force for change', that is, starting up a process of providing better services for carers.

Family doctors (GPs) are now the most important link between families and specialist services. People running specialist services are now encouraged to involve family doctors in care planning and to ensure, at any rate, that they know who service users' care coordinators are, and how to get hold of services in an emergency, particularly out of hours. Recently, the Department of Health has given family doctors the power to remove violent patients from their lists immediately. However, if it is possible that the violence has arisen because of mental illness, the needs of the patient must be dealt with before considering removal from the GP's list. Occasionally people with severe mental illness do get involved in incidents at GP surgeries. It is useful to know that if this makes it impossible for the family doctor to continue caring for the patient, they must, at any rate, arrange for alternative services to meet their needs. It is regarded as good practice for family doctors who feel they must remove someone from their list to inform the Community Mental Health Team before it happens.

Specialist psychiatric services have been given a number of principles for providing care for mentally ill people. Apart from those we have already mentioned, they are encouraged to respect the individual qualities and social, cultural, linguistic and religious background of their clients. As well as taking into account the needs, wishes and convenience, both of clients and of their carers, services are encouraged to give people as much self-determination as possible.

An increasing amount of attention is being given to the role of voluntary organisations in the overall provision of services for people with mental health problems.

Another area where there has been a great deal of development in the last fifteen years has been the contribution of both private and charitable providers of services and care. The last conservative government introduced the idea of the *purchaser provider split*. This split was introduced in order to prevent too cosy a relationship (and, it is argued, a poorer service) between those who needed the service and those who offered it. *Purchasers of care*, at one time the district health authority, would contract with a local provider. The provider of mental health care was usually the local NHS Trust, but in theory it could be a private organization. The idea was that the threat of losing the contract would introduce the beneficial effects of competition and drive up standards. In practice the beneficial effects were few and the increased micromanagement required was not entirely a good thing.

The incoming labour government did not initially use the language of competition in the same way, but the splitting of the selection and delivery of services has continued and the resultant monitoring and the need to justify what has been provided is probably helpful. Services are now commissioned throughout health and social services (the new Primary Care Trusts (PCTs) have a major role in this), and in theory these services are then monitored for quality. Services that do badly can in theory be replaced by a competing service. While this sounds sensible in practice, it does impose a considerable increase in bureaucracy, and care coordinators may spend more time than they did in providing information needed by managers. It often means many forms have to be filled in and various procedures worked through in order for service users to be able to access help with such things as getting back to work, going to college, going to a day centre, befriending or respite care. You will need to talk to your local mental health team for lists of such local services and how they can be accessed.

If your relative is receiving care and treatment in some kind of private or non statutory setting, a hostel for instance, and you think things are going wrong, you should complain. The place to try first is your local Mental Health Team. All NHS Trusts now have standard complaints procedures and all complaints will be investigated by a senior manager. This can of course take some time.

Unfortunately, one of the things that sometimes happens when people with severe mental health problems are living at home is that they may come into contact with the courts. This may be because of some kind of public incident, not necessarily a violent one. However, people who are mentally disordered occasionally commit other petty crimes of various types. If they get arrested as a result, they are quite likely to end up appearing in court. In the past this sometimes meant they were sentenced without proper regard to their mental health needs. Again, the Government has issued guidance recently to people working in the Criminal Justice System on how to work with colleagues in mental health. Most courts now have a liaison scheme to guide those with mental health problems through the legal system, and sometimes to divert them away from it if it seems justice will not be done by proceeding. Even so, it may be difficult to get the psychiatric needs of people with severe mental illness properly considered when they appear in the courts. In such circumstances, you may have to be the first supporter of your relative. This may mean ensuring that lawyers and other court officials know about the mental health problem, as long as your relative agrees with this disclosure.

One of the important developments in the last decade in the attitude of the Government and its agents has been the acceptance that service users' relatives and other carers should be involved as far as possible in the organisation of care. Carers are seen as having a particular role in helping teams to identify the needs of clients, in helping the team keep in touch with them, and encouraging them to keep to their care plans. Indeed, the principle is that carers attend the meeting and should receive a copy of the Care Plan, provided their relative agrees.

The idea of involving relatives and friends of people with health problems is one of the expectations set out in the Patients' Charter. The Department of Health published a framework for local community care charters early in 1996. The key part of this is putting users and carers first. The idea is that local agencies will be committed to involving users and carers in the assessment process and care planning. They must respect users' personal beliefs, show courtesy and respect at all times, and set a high standard in dealing with letters and enquiries. They must also act to protect the confidentiality of information.

Problems often arise when service users refuse to have their relatives involved in their care. If service users are adamant that their family or carers should not be involved, the mental health services are obliged to respect these wishes. There are only a few exceptions. One is where, for example, approved social workers are required by law to inform the nearest relative if someone is being considered for compulsory detention, or has indeed been detained. Another is where public interest outweighs the imperative of confidentiality. This might arise, for instance, if the client was making specific threats which in some way involved the carer.

This brings us on to another important set of guidelines. These are the ones concerned with the protection of information. As might be imagined, there are conflicting requirements. On the one hand, where a number of mental health and social service professionals work together for the good of clients, they need to have the fullest possible information so that their judgements and decisions can be as effective as possible. When people with severe mental health problems are difficult to help, the failure to communicate may lead to real problems, and sometimes tragedies. However, the Government recognises that at the same time people with these problems are entitled to the same confidential handling of information as any other health or social service client.

Information about clients is protected in a number of ways. First, mental health professionals have codes of conduct placing very strict limits on the disclosure on the information. This is backed up by their professional disciplinary organisation. So, for example, a doctor can be severely disciplined by the General Medical Council if he or she breaches patient confidentiality. In addition, information about clients is covered by a well established common law duty of confidence. Finally, if the information is held on a computer, it is specifically protected by the Data Protection Act of 1984. The Government have also adopted a European Union Directive on data protection. One general rule is that information given for one purpose may not be given to a third party or used for a different purpose without the consent of clients. However, this is not a rigid rule. This is because it may sometimes act to the detriment of clients.

Service users and carers should know that personal information may need to pass between health and social service personnel, and people working for other agencies, like probation, housing, or voluntary sectors. Usually this is part of the normal care planning process, and unless service users object, information is given on a 'need-to-know' basis to people with a direct interest. This would include, for instance, somebody employed by a private nursing home. If service users or carers object to this passage of information, it may mean that the whole process of planning care has to be reorganised. In general, the passage of information is on a need-to-know basis, and somebody given information in this way should not pass it on to a third party unless that person is entitled to it. Occasionally information may be passed on without the client's consent, where a history of violence, for example, means that this should be done in the public interest. Occasionally clinical workers may need to take legal advice whether this is permissible.

Service users and people authorised to act on their behalf have statutory rights to know what information is on record about them. Access to computer records in which someone is identified by name is primarily given by the Data Protection Act. However, service users also have the right of access to written records under the Access to Health Records Act 1990. This applies only to records that were made on or after the 1st November 1991. Even then, there are circumstances under which service users may not be entitled to see their records. If the record holder thinks that it would cause serious harm to the physical or mental health of the service user, or to anyone else, they can withhold access. Another circumstance is where the records contain information which relates to, or is provided by, some non professional person, if that person can be identified and has not consented to its disclosure. Although service users do not actually have a right to see any of their records preceding 1991, the record holder may allow them access. Basically, the guiding principle is that service users should be allowed to know what is written about them if at all possible.

Finally, the most recent legislation affecting all NHS Trusts, not just those for mental health services, is a new right for service users to be copied into correspondence about them. This can happen only once the service user has signed a document giving consent to this, which includes consent as to where and how they receive this information. Some service users for example wish to ensure that such information is not delivered to their home address. This is a new policy, and it remains to be seen if it will be useful. So far all service users asked have wished to be copied in, though we have heard, perhaps apocryphally, that once received, disposal of such confidential information is a problem; thus one reported solution was lining the budgie's cage.

Your local mental health services are obliged to have a written policy on access to records which you can ask them for. Usually this would state that if the service user makes a request to see his or her record, this should happen within 21 days from the date of application. Service users can also authorise other people to seek access to health information about them. Obviously, under these circumstances, staff must make absolutely sure that the other person really is acting at the request of the service user.

4 Services

THE PEOPLE INVOLVED IN THE CARE OF YOUR RELATIVE

As described in chapter 3, mental health services are currently organised in multidisciplinary teams. Nowadays these are likely to include a team leader (who will usually be a senior community psychiatric nurse), a senior social worker, a consultant psychiatrist, and a variety of other members, from disciplines, such as occupational therapy, community psychiatric nursing, clinical psychology, social work and psychiatry. The team will usually designate two or three people to become involved in the care of your relative. One of these will be your relative's care coordinator (see Ch. 3). A care coordinator may be from any discipline, a community psychiatric nurse (CPN), a social worker, an occupational therapist, senior house officer, or clinical psychologist, depending on your relative's particular problems, so it may sometimes seem as though the consultant never sees them. The team however meet regularly to discuss the progress of each client and if your relative is on the CPA (see Ch. 3) they have by law to be discussed (reviewed) at least every six months. However, people sometimes feel that although they were 'under Doctor Smith', they were only seen once or twice, so the doctor could not have known much about them. If the team is working properly, this will not be true, because each member will keep the others informed. The main advantage of this team approach is that clients are seen as a whole person, who may have needs that are best satisfied by a particular member of the team, not necessarily a psychiatrist. It also means that you do not just have to rely on one member of staff, who may be unavailable or with whom you may disagree. The disadvantage is that you may feel you never get to talk to the same person, and sometimes none of them may seem to know what is happening! This can be a real problem, particularly in a crisis, but a good team will try not to let it happen often.

Although many people do not realise it, psychiatrists have to train as ordinary medical doctors first. This usually takes up to five or six years. In this country, they then have to undertake a further six years or so of training in psychiatry. After about three years of this time, they will sit the entrance examination for membership of the Royal College of Psychiatrists. If they pass, they are entitled to put 'MRCPsych' after their names, initials you may have seen, for instance, in correspondence. After a further period of supervised work, they may apply for posts as consultants.

Clearly, this is a long training; sad to say, some service users and their relatives have felt it must have missed the point, creating psychiatrists who did not seem very good at offering support and information. Things do appear to have improved over the last decade or so, following more emphasis on these aspects during training.

Consultants Psychiatrists are assisted by junior doctors who are part way through their training: there are two categories: Specialist Grade Registrars (SpRs), and Senior House Officers (SHOs).

One popular image of psychiatrists, perhaps the most popular one, is of someone very powerful who behaves rather oddly and has an uncanny ability to see into the deep recesses of the mind. The truth is more down to earth. A good psychiatrist may have insights into a situation that you may not have thought of, but this comes from experience and an objective alertness to all the possibilities. Psychiatrists need information to do this, and this is why assessment involves so many questions (see page 82). They may be better at detecting false information than untrained people but they are still far from infallible. One of us (Paul) is a consultant psychiatrist:-

Until recently, I worked with three teams. One was located on a general psychiatric ward. It included psychiatric nurses of different grades, an occupational therapist and a senior house officer. The beds on the ward were always full – indeed in our unit bed occupation was said to run at over 110%. This did not mean people shared beds, but that beds for people who were on leave from the ward, or beds in the private sector were used to cope with the overflow of patients. The second team was a community mental health team. This had a team base outside the hospital. It included community psychiatric nurses and an occupational therapist. The two teams also shared a specialist grade registrar, and a clinical psychologist. Between them they were responsible for an area of inner London with a population of 38,000.

As I am primarily an academic psychiatrist, and also have managerial and administrative responsibilities, I 'job-shared' this National Health Service work with a colleague. Two of my sessions were team meetings on the ward. People with fairly severe episodes of mental disorder were admitted to the ward, where they were assessed by the various members of the team. In the team meeting I heard about these new patients and saw them, and the team came to conclusions about diagnosis, treatment and management that would best help the patient. In this I operated a bit like the chairman of a committee, summing up the consensus view of my colleagues. For some purposes, as responsible medical officer, I was supposed to have the final word, but decisions were almost always by joint agreement.

I also heard about the progress of patients admitted earlier, but never had time to see more than a few of them each week. However, I did see them at Care Programme Approach meetings, which is when important decisions are made, for instance, about discharge arrangements or an application for supported accommodation. Sometimes I saw the patients' relatives, although that was also done by other members of the team. Some of my time was used to teach and supervise my junior colleagues, who were responsible for the everyday medical input in the ward, and also did some outpatient and community work. This is an efficient way of using limited resources. This pattern of working is a common one, repeated in wards and clinics throughout Britain. Some consultants also run outpatient clinics in general practice health centres, a trend which is increasing.

I worked in these teams for about eight years, before moving to other responsibilities a couple of years ago. In that time there were many improvements – beds became less crowded, and the community and ward aspects of the work became better integrated. Moreover, the local Trust was responsible for introducing improved ways of working and set up specialist teams to deal with particularly difficult problems. The most successful of these was the introduction of a crisis resolution team, which had the remit of liaising closely and widely, particularly with the community mental health teams, the ward teams, local GPs, service users and carers. The purpose was to try and ensure a rapid response if someone appeared to be relapsing or developing some other type of crisis related to their mental health problems. This had the aim of avoiding hospital admission if at all possible, and the team was quite successful in this. I provided one session a week to this team, which involved providing advice but also sometimes visiting people at home, assessing exactly what their needs might be, and working out how to meet them (see below for a fuller description of how they work).

Recently I moved out of what might be seen as mainstream mental health work because our Trust took on responsibility for the mental health service in the two prisons that happen to lie in our catchment area. So I now provide sessions to this new service, where many of the inmates have very serious mental health problems.

Nurses are also organised in various grades. The head nurse in a ward is sometimes called the 'Ward Manager'. After psychiatric training lasting three years, nurses become Registered Mental Nurses (RMN). Some mental health nurses are also State Registered Nurses (SRN), that is, they have a general nursing qualification, and these days many have taken degrees in nursing or related subjects.

Mental health nurses do still work in hospital wards and clinics. However, these days a majority of nurses, the so-called Community Psychiatric Nurses (CPNs), spend their time visiting patients in their homes. They have all had long experience of psychiatric nursing, often as ward managers. They will also have undertaken training courses in community psychiatry. Such nurses usually have their base in a community mental health centre, although a few work directly with family doctors. They are closely involved in the treatment of people who have been discharged from hospital following serious episodes of mental illness. They also care for people who may not go into hospital very frequently, but who have persistent problems in managing their lives because of their mental health difficulties. They keep an eye on their clients' medication and may give injections. They monitor the general situation of clients and their families, and provide a significant source of advice and support. They also keep the other members of the Community Mental Health Team informed of progress, so they provide an important channel of communication.

John has been a community psychiatric nurse (CPN) for about three years. During most of this time he has been visiting Phil, as his Care Coordinator. Phil is a young man about John's own age who suffers from schizophrenia. He has been reasonably well, and able to live at home with his parents. There are rarely any problems, but sometimes Phil's parents like to be able to talk things over with John, which he is always ready to do. Indeed he has become something of a friend to all the family. He also gives Phil a long acting injection every three weeks. Recently Phil began to experience a return of some disturbing symptoms but with John's help, he and his family were able to cope with this and things settled down again. The enduring relationship that has developed between John and Phil and his family is a good example of the valuable role of many community psychiatric nurses in helping people manage the problems of a serious mental illness.

Social workers also have a considerable role in psychiatry and these days are part of the team. They too will be Care coordinators, involved with individual patients, offering support and counselling, and using a range of techniques aimed at improving the patient's ability to cope. They also have expert knowledge about welfare rights, practical aids and community facilities. Some of them have had further training and have particular powers and duties under the Mental Health Act which means they are an approved social worker or ASW, and can section people if necessary for their safety or that of others.

Clinical psychologists have a degree in psychology, following which they undergo a further three-year specialist clinical training. This training now leads to a doctorate in clinical psychology. Some have also done another research based degree after a period of research (a PhD). Both of these routes mean that they are called 'Doctor', so that this title is not confined to those with medical training. You may perhaps have been confused by this, not being sure if the person you are talking to is a doctor of the medical sort or has a different expertise.

Clinical Psychologists specialise in assessing and treating psychological problems of all kinds. They also have an interest in measuring and evaluating peoples' progress. Clinical psychology is still a relatively small profession, although very much a growth area. Its members are normally based in mental health teams, some work in community health centres, with GPs, or in general hospitals. One of us, Elizabeth, is a consultant clinical psychologist:-

I work with a multidisciplinary team which specialises in providing continuing care for people in the local area with severe adult mental health problems. Members of our team are linked in with our local GP practices, and service users are seen in their homes, at a local drop-in centre, in a GP practice or in our team base around the side of the Maudsley Hospital. We have a few beds in a local ward for those that require admission; these are always full. We receive referrals mainly from another team, which does initial assessment and 'brief treatment' for those with less severe mental health problems, or from other teams telling us that someone has moved into our area and we need to take over their care.

As I work in a deprived inner London area, with 40% of service users coming from a variety of ethnic minorities, the problems we have to deal with can be very diverse and sometimes alarming, ranging from someone being attacked or evicted, or needing help from housing or physical health agencies because of a multitude of overlapping difficulties. I see around 10 service users in a weekly clinic, and have a particular interest in those with long-term psychosis. Psychologists are specialists in cognitive behavioural treatments, which means talking to people both about what they think (cognition) and what they do (behaviour), and trying to help them change negative thought patterns or unhelpful behaviour patterns that can make anxiety, depression or psychosis more problematic. Psychologists do not administer drug treatments, (the psychiatrists in the team are asked to monitor and advise on this). Instead they offer 'talking' therapies to individuals, carers and groups, discuss the particular psychological problems of other care coordinators clients, and help the team review care plans for everyone on the team's case load.

Separately, I am Director of a specialist clinic at the Maudsley which offers cognitive behavioural treatments (CBT) to those with psychosis or related problems. These people are referred from the local area, and from the rest of London and the surrounding boroughs; it relies on people attending for outpatient appointments. We see about 50 people a year for at least 6 months of CBT for psychosis, if they will attend. Many people are seen for longer than this, but often less frequently.

I have a research interest in developing CBT for psychosis. I have also done research into family work for psychosis, offering help to relatives who look after a mentally ill family member, and in how best to offer help to carers. At the moment I supervise care coordinators and other staff who do local family work for psychosis. With colleagues, I have written books about both of these psychological treatments (see Appendix).

Both CBT for psychosis and family intervention for psychosis have been recommended by the National Institute for Clinical Excellence (NICE) guidelines for treatment of schizophrenia. NICE recommends evidence-based treatments if they are effective. This means that both of these psychological treatments are being implemented in NHS Trusts at the moment. Although not widely available, the plan is that this should improve.

Occupational therapists undergo a three year course of training. Their job is to design and carry out programmes of activities intended to overcome difficulties and to foster or maintain a better quality of life. They are particularly interested in helping people to improve leisure and job-related skills. These activities may be based in a hospital ward, in an Occupational Therapy department, or in the community where most occupational therapists are now based, acting as care coordinaters like the rest of the team. Unfortunately, despite their skills, there is a huge shortage of OT at the moment, and many teams no longer have access to them.

There is, in practice, a lot of overlap in what members of these professions do when they see service users. Much of the assessment and treatment of mental health problems is carried out by getting to know patients and by talking to them over a considerable period of time. Each profession has its own particular specialist knowledge as well. Only psychiatrists, (because of their medical qualification) are able to prescribe medication at the moment. This is why service users are often particularly encouraged to 'see the Doctor'. Mental health services are usually organised in teams because this is a good way to use the different contributions that each profession can make. Occasionally there are disadvantages. If the team is badly organised, there may be failures of communication. Each member of the team may think that someone else is dealing with a particular problem, when in fact no-one is. If there is a possibility that this has happened in the case of your relative, you should raise the matter with your care coordinator, the person on the team you have had most contact with, or the team manager. However, a good team should be one of your most useful supports.

THE SERVICES AVAILABLE TO YOUR RELATIVE

For the majority of people who become mentally ill, the professional they see first is their General Practitioner (GP), sometimes called the family practitioner or family doctor. They will usually be seen, by appointment or on spec, in the GP's surgery, although sometimes GPs will make a home visit, if a surgery appointment is not feasible. They normally deal with minor cases themselves, but will refer more serious conditions to the local mental health team. This is sometimes done by making an outpatient appointment for your relation to see a psychiatrist. This may take place at your local general or psychiatric hospital, although many psychiatrists these days have their out-patient sessions in community resource centres, and a few in health centres. If an out-patient appointment is made for your mentally ill relative, you should be aware that there is likely to be some delay, a few weeks perhaps, before they are seen. Psychiatrists like their patients to be accompanied to appointments, partly so that they have a further source of information if they need it. Do not be reticent about asking to see the psychiatrist if they do not themselves suggest it, or about seeking answers to your queries. Your relative may have to wait for some time, particularly if they are seen first by the SHO who will then discuss things with the Consultant. Going with them to the appointment will give them some company while they wait, and this may be especially appreciated if they feel apprehensive about it. Another route to the psychiatric team is to be seen first by any of its members, who will do an initial assessment, and then discuss with the rest of the team what services the person needs.

Sometimes more urgent action seems necessary, and your GP will arrange for a home visit whereby the psychiatrist or another member of the multidisciplinary team will come to your home and assess your relative there. This can usually be arranged within a few days.

Mental health professionals assess patients largely by collecting information, both from the person themselves and from their relatives, and even occasionally from other acquaintances. They do this in order to discover what form the problem takes, what sort of person the individual normally is, and what stresses and strains they have been exposed to. The psychiatrist will usually obtain informa-tion about your relative's symptoms directly from them, but may back this up by getting an account from you or other members of the family. A service user's relations will often be the best people to describe the way problems have developed. In addition, the psychiatrist will gather background information to provide the overall context within which the origins of the disorder can be understood. This means they may well have information provided by your family doctor.

Nowadays, in many areas, such assessments are carried out by members of a community mental health team, at a community resource centre of some kind, or by visiting your relative at home. Obviously, it is very important that the information you give to members of the mental health team is as true and as full as possible. Sometimes, you may feel that a question is irrelevant or intrusive. You might then prefer not to answer it fully. However covering things up in this way may hinder the clinical staff from understanding problems properly.

Very occasionally, schizophrenia or bipolar disorder can be mimicked by bodily diseases. The psychiatrist may order blood tests, and occasionally other investigations like a brain scan, to exclude these, either as a routine or as a result of symptoms that suggest they are appropriate.

After clients have been assessed, GPs will often carry on the treatment of minor conditions. More serious problems may involve regular monitoring. However, a service user will sometimes need to be admitted to hospital. These days, it is understood that most people find hospital admission (to a mental hospital), frightening and difficult and would prefer to stay in their own homes. Most areas therefore now have a system whereby anyone being considered for admission is seen and assessed by a member of a specialist team for their suitability for home treatment. These teams have various names, crisis intervention (CI) or crisis resolution (CR) will usually figure in the acronym. They will again be multidisciplinary, but usually consist of psychiatrists and community mental health nurses. They aim to provide intensive home visiting, sometimes several times a day, to ensure that an individual can stay safely at home. Such teams usually do this for 2 or 3 weeks, until the crisis has passed. The individual's care will then be handed back to the original local team. These home treatment teams are meant to be equivalent to a hospital stay, which they are set up to try and avoid. They have the same sorts of procedures, including a discharge meeting that you should be involved in (see below). They typically focus on medication resumption and monitoring, and on problem solving around urgent practical difficulties.

However if home treatment is not felt to be suitable, hospital admission will be offered. This will usually be in a local ward in a general hospital or local mental hospital. Many such wards were purpose-built, although some decades ago now, and they are beginning to show their age. They sometimes have a more institutional look than we would prefer these days. In some cases they may be an awkwardly placed ward or even a hospital block originally built for some other purpose and later adapted. A few areas still have their admission wards in old style mental hospitals, although almost all of these have now closed. Many of them were built in Victorian times and served large areas. For this reason they may be quite a long way from your home and difficult to get to.

However they are organised, mental inpatient wards can be noisy, busy and difficult places to feel comfortable in. Sometimes in our inner cities, people stay only a few days and are then transferred to another ward because of bed shortages. It can all be quite confusing. At present there is a lot of emphasis on 'improving ward atmosphere'. Hopefully this will improve things.

If there are no beds available in your local hospital, your relative may be sent for a few days into private care; this is usually in the same city, but very occasionally a whole area will not have a bed and your relative may be placed further away. It was not unknown for a patient from London to be admitted, for example, to a hospital in Leicester, although such extremes are quite unusual these days. Usually admission to a private bed will only be for a few days: it has to be paid for by the NHS and can cost several hundred pounds a night, so local services try not to use them for long.

Virtually all the old style 'long-stay' wards have now closed down. However, some people still need continuing 24 hour care. Under the current guidelines and legislation relating to community care, such people are given a needs assessment (see page 68) by a mental health team member, and then offered a place in a 'high support' hostel in the local area. They no longer stay in hospital for months or years as they used to. A small minority of patients may be so disturbed for so long that they need to live in a secure unit, but even for them the arrangement is not usually permanent.

In psychiatric wards, unlike most medical wards, people have their own clothes and night clothes, so if your relative is being admitted, they will need to take these with them or you will have to bring them along later. They will be received into the ward by the nursing staff who will register them by taking some personal details. Usually after they have settled in the ward, perhaps an hour or two later, they will be visited by a junior psychiatrist who will make a physical examination, record your relative's mental condition, and set in motion some basic physical investigations. They may provide temporary medication for calming your relative down or to help them sleep. Each client has a 'named nurse', who has special responsibility for them and coordinates most aspects of their care. There has recently been a government policy of moving towards single sex wards. It has been felt that mixed wards are too unsafe for women. However, in practice the policy is quite hard to implement, and there can be a considerable cost consequences: thus male patients may have to be sent to the private sector, while beds remain empty on a female-only ward. There are sometimes other unexpected consequences, for instance a reduction in the proportion of women in wards that have not become single sex. This makes them seem even more insecure.

Sleeping accommodation in hospital is usually either in single rooms, or in rooms shared with from two to six other patients. New facilities no longer have dormitory arrangements, so single rooms are becoming increasingly the rule. Most hospitals do have one or two wards which are kept locked, but these are reserved for the most difficult patients, for instance those felt likely to commit suicide or to abscond while seriously unwell. A few hospitals have special mother-and-baby units for those with postnatal psychosis. This permits a mentally ill mother to take some part in caring for her new baby at this important time.

After a few days, your relative's case will be considered in a team or management meeting, still sometimes called a ward round, although this is a term borrowed from hospitals that treat physical illnesses. The consultant psychiatrist usually chairs this, and there are often quite a number of people there, representing the various clinical professions. This can be intimidating for your relative, and may be equally upsetting for you if you have been invited along. However, staff in these meeting are bound by rules of confidentiality, and are there to provide a service for you and your relative. Sometimes, if your relative is likely to be very upset by being seen in the team meeting, a few members of the team may come out to see them more privately.

Most service users admitted from their homes to psychiatric wards will return home when they are discharged. Ideally, discharge should be planned to take place in a gradual manner: it may be suggested at first that your relative returns home perhaps for an afternoon. They may then spend part or all of a weekend at home, and if this seems to go all right, they may then be discharged. This pattern can be varied to suit the needs of individuals and their relatives. However, because hospital beds are now scarce, most admissions to hospital are only for a few weeks and it is not always possible to be as flexible as one would wish. During this process it is important that you keep the clinical staff informed about how things have gone, and what you think the next step should be.

Under the Community Care Act, a patient with severe mental illness cannot be discharged from hospital without a proper discharge plan signed by the consultant and another mental health professional, and agreed by the service user and carer if there is one. This discharge planning meeting (still sometimes called a 'Section 117 meeting' after the part of the Mental Health Act that describes it) is a legal requirement, and you should both be consulted and present at it. This is so that you know of and agree any discharge plans that are made with the team about your relative's care after they leave hospital.

Sometimes, supported accommodation may seem a better option than going home. There are a number of possibilities, including supervised high support hostels, low support hostels, or flats, group homes and supervised lodgings.

Hostels provide for a number of people. They may be set up either by the statutory authorities or by charitable organisations. They vary enormously: some are just places to eat and sleep, others have much more in the way of supervision. Some provide long term accommodation, whereas others are seen very much as staging posts in a full return to life in the community. In some, supervision is quite intensive, with night staff, organised daytime activities, and another set of key-workers/care coordinators. The aim is to place people in the facility that best suits their problems, although this may not always be available.

Group homes are less common these days. They were usually set up in large converted houses. There may be from four to twenty patients living in them. They tended to be provided when the old mental hospitals closed down, and are not so popular now. After the settling in period, they are not heavily supervised, although various members of the mental health team may pop in from time to time. In most ways they try to be like a hostel. The residents have their own rooms, but will share other facilities. They have to work out amongst themselves who does what in the important matters of cooking and cleaning. Some will go out to work or to day centres during the day. In some homes, there is a limit to the length of time someone can live there. Obviously, you and your relative must know about this.

Each local authority has a responsibility to provide accommodation for people leaving psychiatric hospitals if it is needed, provided they previously lived within their boundaries. This accommodation may be in another area, although the first authority will sponsor people to live in it through a financial arrangement with the second. This system has been misused in the past by local authorities in large cities sponsoring discharged mental patients to live in suburban areas or seaside resorts where they have no local links. This happened because there were too few resources locally, but placed a heavy burden on the services in the area where the clients ended up. Many local authorities and voluntary organisations provide sheltered flats and bed-sitters. The accommodation may be purpose built, or a number of flats in a block may be given over to people recovering their mental health. Some support is given, sometimes by social workers or housing officers, sometimes by voluntary sector helpers.

A variety of charitable organisations are involved in the creation of accommodation for former hospital patients. These include the Richmond Fellowship, and several local branches of Mind. A lot of housing associations also provide 'special needs' accommodation that can also be used for those with mental health problems.

The decision for a person to move from home into one of these facilities should be a joint one by them, the relatives they live with, and the clinical team.

People who have longstanding psychiatric problems may require particular services to rehabilitate them. This means helping them to get started again after having been mentally ill. It may include relearning old skills, such as working to a routine, or acquiring new skills, as required for some particular job, or new interests such as painting or pottery. It may also mean helping individuals to regain the confidence needed to go back out into the community. It is usually a very gradual process, certainly not one that can be hurried, so that staff may see it in terms of months or years, particularly for someone who has had several episodes.

Many rehabilitation services provide a work environment. They include facilities specially designed to help those with mental health problems, but some are more general and available to other members of the public. These days most of these sheltered workshops are provided by local charities, although they may be paid for out of social services budgets.

Many mental health services include a day hospital. People attend this during the day from their homes, and the emphasis is very much on rehabilitation. Occasionally, the day hospital may be seen as an alternative to full time admission, but usually it is used by recently discharged patients. It will often have its own occupational therapy and sheltered workshops. The principles of sheltered work are described in more detail below. It may be a good idea for you to ask about the local facilities available for those recovering from severe mental illness as they vary considerably around the country. It is probably best to ask the local mental health team when they do a needs assessment, but your care coordinator or GP (family doctor) should also know what is available.

There are also day centres. These are usually provided by voluntary or charitable organisations. Your local team should have a list of facilities like this in your area.

When we first started to work in mental health, a normal aim of treatment and rehabilitation was for individuals to return to full time employment. Even now, people who suffer from the more minor psychiatric disorders assume that they will go back to their job when they are better. However, times have changed for those who become more seriously ill, particularly with a disorder like schizophrenia, which can impair performance even when the more acute symptoms have abated. Many either never return to outside employment, or have infrequent temporary jobs. The figures of a recent survey across the European Union showed that 80% of people with schizophrenia remained unemployed afterwards.

Nevertheless, there are facilities geared towards helping people return to some employment, even if part time or sheltered. They are based on the premise that this may be a long process. Most are now run by voluntary agencies. Attendance may involve getting back into a previous work routine, for instance factory or clerical work, or retraining for some new occupation.

The facilities most often used now to help people recover from mental health problems include job clubs, job agencies geared to those with previous mental health problems, and a whole range of college or leisure based courses.

Organisations that provide employment include the Richmond Fellowship, and some local branches of Mind, and RETHINK. As well as helping people to recover lost skills, and to learn new ones, these organisations provide guidance about many aspects of the return to open employment. However, it may be that your relative never makes the transfer to a job in the outside world. Sheltered employment may then become a reasonable and rewarding option.

Many people who have recovered from a mental illness and are returning to the hurly burly of the employment market will initially need additional help. This can be obtained from the Disablement Resettlement Officer (DRO) who works in your local Job Centre. The DRO can give you help and advice on job opportunities, employment training, specialist schemes to help people with disabilities, and the Disabled Persons Employment Register. In this country any firm that employs more than 20 people must reserve 3% of its posts for persons who are registered as disabled. This may help your relative in getting a job – it is the DRO's responsibility to consider placing someone on the Disabled Person's Register. However, there is still often a long waiting list, and people sometimes feel unduly stigmatised by this.

Sometimes it may be possible for your relative to get practical guidance on the frequently harrowing business of attending job interviews. This may be provided by professionals from the organisation that is helping to get them back into employment, or by attending a job club provided by a local charity.

People who become mentally ill may lose their job. However, mental illness on its own is not grounds for dismissal. If your relative's employer wanted to dismiss them, they would need to ask your relative to provide a medical report concerning their fitness to work. If the doctor providing the report was of the opinion that your relative would not be able to work again for a year, the employer would then be in a position to dismiss them. They could also dismiss them for poor performance at work if this was apparent. However, the employer cannot dismiss someone for either of these reasons without giving warning, and your relative has in any case the right to appeal to an industrial tribunal if they do so within three months. Mind's legal advice department (see web site) can advise them or you about the legal position over dismissal on grounds of mental illness.

DEALING WITH MENTAL HEALTH PROFESSIONALS

If you live with someone who has had a severe mental illness, it almost inevitably means that you will come into close and perhaps frequent contact with mental health staff. In the past, these relationships were often uncomfortable for both sides, and this can sometimes still be the case. This may make obtaining treatment or help for your relative or for yourself more difficult than it need be, and it may even impair their progress. It is extremely important that you should try not to be intimidated in your interviews with staff. Similarly it is useful if you try not to antagonise them. Do not be dissuaded from asking any questions you want to, or from expressing concern over what worries you, but be aware that they are usually trying their best in overstretched and sometimes badly funded services.

Often, these staff-relative relationships start badly because of an upsetting hospital admission, which relatives, service users and even staff may afterwards feel has not been handled properly. If your first introduction to the local mental health facilities involved following your screaming relative down a corridor late at night accompanied by police, this will make subsequent relationships difficult. Such scenes are fairly rare, but if someone has developed a serious mental illness and is unwilling to be seen by a psychiatrist, or refuses to go to hospital, they may be sectioned under the Mental Health Act (see Chapter 5). The result may be a crisis and there may be violence. At this stage the police are likely to be involved. This can all be extremely unpleasant and shocking for everyone. Sometimes, such crises happen very suddenly and are quite unavoidable, but it is natural to want to blame someone, and clinical staff may be a convenient, and sometimes justified, target.

After your relative has been admitted, staff will usually want to ask you many questions about their early history, the existence of problems in the past and intimate details of their relationships, and sometimes, if it is relevant, yours too. The clinical staff see it as necessary to obtain the maximum amount of information about their clients as quickly as possible after an admission, and relatives are normally the best people to provide this. However, relatives often feel that these questions are unnecessarily intrusive and endlessly repeated. They may also think the situation is unfairly one-sided, as their own questions and queries are not answered. To an extent, this situation arises because the psychiatric team is, quite properly, careful about not jumping to conclusions and uses detailed information and observation to shape decisions. However, even these days some professionals have particular difficulties in talking openly with relatives. This is of course crazy – if a mental health professional cannot feel easy in talking to people, who can? – but, as we say, it is still sometimes the case. Some professionals still have particular difficulties in admitting that they do not know the answer to a given question, though relatives have a right to know if this is so.

The staff's assessment of a patient, of what treatment will be best, and of how someone will respond to it, usually takes some time to complete, and it may indeed continue to change as more information becomes available. This delay can be frustrating for you as a relative: the psychiatric team will often hesitate after admission or initial assessment before deciding on the best treatments for someone. Even then, they may be hesitant or even evasive about telling you of these decisions. These days it should at least have been made clear within the team who is responsible for saying what to whom. Nevertheless it may still be quite hard for you to get from staff any authoritative statement about what is wrong with your relative. Instant answers to insistent questions may not be available. Staff may not know the answers, or may be reluctant to tell relatives and risk upsetting them by being too pessimistic. Unfortunately, it is impossible to be sure about the likely course of a severe episode of mental illness, and this may account for some of the reticence that relatives encounter. While we know that some patients will recover completely, it is rarely possible at the outset to recognise who will recover and who will have continuing problems. Staff may deal with this by being imprecise. However, more general information should be available, and you can and should ask for it.

If you feel you are still not getting the information you need, you must make this plain to the staff, particularly as they now have a clear duty to keep you informed and involved. It is perfectly reasonable for you to ask to speak to the consultant psychiatrist or other members of the clinical team to discuss their views on your relative's problems, the sorts of treatments that are available, what can be expected on their return home, the team's opinion on the sort of mental illness it is, and how your relative is recovering from it.

It is often useful to have more than one appointment with staff, as it may be impossible for you to ask all your questions and remember the answers during in an initial interview. Do not be afraid to take a notebook to write down what you are being told, or to ask for explanations if difficult technical terms are used. You should not hide the fact of your visit from your relative (it is after all perfectly reasonable for you to want to find out as much as possible about their problems), but how much you discuss what was said will depend on the exact circumstances.

Not all the problems of getting information are due to the uncertainty of the situation or the inadequacies of staff. It is possible to be told a thing and not really take it on board, especially if the experience is novel and you are distressed by it. It usually takes time, much more time than with a more straightforward physical illness, for carers to take in exactly what is happening to their relative. It may be many months before you come to an understanding of some of the causes (which even the staff may be unsure of) and become able to accept some of the long term implications of a severe mental illness, both for your relative and for the family as a whole.

You are likely to experience a range of emotions at this difficult time. You may feel that staff do not consult you over treatment decisions, or give you adequate support, and even that they are blaming you for your relative's problems. You may well feel very confused and worried about the future. It is usually a great relief that someone else is now trying to help, but such feelings may also make you feel very guilty. Other feelings that people in your position have described include those of inadequacy, hopelessness, bitterness that these things have happened at all, and great upset that the patient has become so unwell and vulnerable. It is not surprising that the attempts of staff and relatives to communicate with each other at this time are often unsuccessful.

Many find self-help groups provide a useful place where carers can obtain information and exchange experiences. One organisation that offers this sort of a forum is RETHINK. Talking to relatives who have been through it all before can be a great help to you if you are going through a bad patch. You in turn may be able to help others at a later date.

SECOND OPINIONS

In the National Health Service, it is accepted that people will sometimes want an opinion from another doctor. If your relative wants such a second opinion, they must find a doctor willing to examine them, and there is no obligation on any given doctor to do this. In general, the doctor in charge of their case will be agreeable to them seeking a second opinion and there will be no difficulty in doing so. Your relative may do this entirely through your family doctor, but if they themselves discover a psychiatrist willing to see them, the family doctor will probably agree to make a formal referral for them.

There may occasionally be particular problems for psychiatric patients who want to be referred for the opinion of another doctor. Mental health services are responsible for all the people living in a particular area, linked to GP practices within their catchment areas. These are usually rigidly observed, the so called treatment by postcode. It may therefore be difficult to obtain the opinion of a doctor working in a mental health service that deals with another area. The doctors attached to a given service are likely to work closely together and the client may feel, with some justification, that a second opinion from a close colleague of their own doctor might be prejudiced. The psychiatrist may also be tempted to feel that clients' reluctance to accept a first opinion is due to their psychiatric state.

The situation for the mentally ill is therefore sometimes unsatisfactory. One way round the problem is to seek a second opinion from a psychiatrist in a service connected to a medical school (a Teaching Trust). There will usually be at least one of these in any large city. The services that teaching trusts provide are not usually restricted to their catchment area. The disadvantage of this method of obtaining a second opinion is that it may involve travelling quite a distance. Your Family Doctor can make the referral, although it is useful if your or your relative can supply the name of a doctor you would like to consult at the hospital. However, the Royal College of Psychiatrists makes it a rule not to give out the names of suitable psychiatrists, so you would have to do some work to find a name for yourself.

It is possible to seek a further opinion privately, that is, outside the National Health Service. You and your relative will be responsible for the fee for this opinion. Your doctor may know a psychiatrist who sees patients in this way. Any long term private medical treatment is very expensive indeed, particularly if it involves frequent hospital in-patient treatment, but you may feel that an appointment for a second opinion is worth paying for if it sets your mind at rest. Private medical insurance schemes are unlikely to cover long-term psychiatric care.

Detained patients have the right to a second opinion under the Mental Health Act: the Mental Health Act Commission has the duty of appointing a doctor to provide this second opinion.

We have given advice on how you can best set about obtaining what you need for your relative and yourself from the psychiatric services. There are, however, still many places in this country where local facilities are under-funded or underdeveloped, or where the local professionals are apathetic, ignorant, unsympathetic or just plain overworked. Sometimes, through great efforts, you may be able to browbeat them into extending the provision they offer to you and your relative. In some circumstances, no adequate service is forthcoming, try as you might, and you may have to turn more towards independent organisations, such as RETHINK or Mind. Such organisations offer information and support, but they can often also exert pressure on services to develop local facilities, or be more responsive to your needs.

There are now advocacy services available for clients, if they feel services are inadequate. These are usually linked in to mental health services, and the local trust administration, or again social services, your team or your family doctor should be able to advise you how to ask them to act for you to elicit what you or your relative feel is a reasonable service. If all else fails, each health service trust now has to make clear what their complaints procedure is, and it should be easy to find out how to do this. Once a complaint has been made, a Hospital Trust has to respond, investigate it and reply. If you are still not satisfied, your local MP can take up a particular incident on your behalf, if they are also persuaded that there is a case to answer.

5   Treatment

Several treatments are offered routinely for severe mental illness in NHS mental health services in all parts of the country. These may include admission to hospital, or intensive home treatment, physical treatments like medication, and various psychological and social treatments. They are all described below. Private medical care tends to offer a similar approach.

ADMISSION TO HOSPITAL AND INTENSIVE HOME TREATMENT

If your relative has just become unwell with severe depression, mania or schizophrenia, they are likely to be offered either hospital admission or home treatment. Intensive home treatment means that people are visited, sometimes several times a day for help with medication and problem solving of urgent practical problems (as discussed in Ch. 4). This is because it has been recognised that most people dislike being admitted to a mental hospital, and would prefer to stay at home. Beds in hospital are expensive as well as unpopular, and continue to be cut back in order to try and help people stay at home. As a result there are fewer mental health beds in NHS facilities than ever, and getting admitted to hospital may in fact be a last resort.

In principle, admission to hospital is an attempt to treat problems away from the home environment, either because the person cannot or will not stay at home, or because they are refusing treatment there. Admission to a psychiatric ward can be a way of reducing the likelihood of life threatening suicide attempts for instance. However, it is rarely offered just for this reason. It is mainly an attempt to calm things down, in a more neutral and closely observed situation, where staff can get a better picture of what the difficulties are. At its best a hospital admission provides rest, shelter and a neutral environment in which to assess calmly and begin to treat difficulties. This is meant to reduce problems. In reality some wards are overcrowded, noisy, and at times violent. They can be difficult and frightening places to be admitted to or to visit. Wards are usually full, with people being admitted and discharged at a high rate. They take people in who are quite disturbed, and who may be dishevelled and confused. As a result it can be very difficult to prevent psychiatric wards from looking dirty, shabby and rather dreary. Despite staff efforts to improve ward atmosphere and the facilities offered, it can be an uphill struggle to maintain a calm and pleasant environment. This is partly why an admission to hospital can be such a shock for both yourselves and your relative. It is easy to see why home treatment is often preferred both by staff and service users. However, home treatment can have disadvantages. One is that instead of service users having a few days in hospital, so that you can both have some respite from your difficulties, home treatment means that although things calm down, your level of anxiety and upset may remain high. Although home treatment is meant to be equivalent to a hospital admission, in its effectiveness, and in its intensity, it will not always feel equivalent.

If someone has been advised to have an admission for treatment, but refuses, it may be decided that it is in their best interest to be admitted 'under a section', that is, without their consent through the powers of the Mental Health Act (see page 146). While relatives usually see the necessity of compulsory admission, they and the service user may be understandably distressed. Some may be left feeling very guilty, as if they have 'betrayed' the patient.

Psychiatric hospitals, and mental illness itself, are seen as frightening or shameful by many people. Most people do not ever visit a psychiatric ward until they have to. There is often an image, unfortunately confirmed by the more lurid films and TV programmes, (such as 'One flew over a cuckoo's nest') that once you enter a psychiatric hospital it is difficult to get out again, and that the people there are bizarre and terrifying. The reality is more mundane. Mental hospitals have changed considerably, and very few of the older hospitals still exist. Ironically, many of them have been turned into desirable residential properties with luxurious apartments. Most have been replaced by purpose-built or newly adapted units. Nevertheless, some psychiatric wards are still located in buildings that retain a forbidding exterior or an isolated position, and this can take some time to get used to. Psychiatric facilities are now frequently based in General Hospitals, and this may make an admission easier to accept and more convenient. When it is not the first time a patient has been admitted, both relative and patients will know more of what they have to deal with.

You may find it hard to visit your relative in hospital, perhaps because of practical inconvenience, perhaps because you don't really relish the ward environment. Nevertheless, they will very probably set great store by your visits, so try to go as often as possible. Apart from the requirements of ward activities like OT (see page), visiting is usually fairly unrestricted. When you visit, it will normally be all right to go for a walk or out to a local café with your relative, although you should tell the nursing staff what you are doing and when you will be back.

'PHYSICAL' TREATMENT

Drugs in mental illness

Effective treatments in psychiatry are of fairly recent date. Before the 1950s, psychiatrists had little to offer their patients except sedation and nursing care. If people got better, it was usually the result of the natural ebb and flow of their illness. However, around that time there were a number of innovations, including the first drugs effective against schizophrenia and depression, and the development of techniques of rehabilitation. Retired clinicians who can remember those times will say how dramatic the effect of introducing these new treatments really was. It became possible to get enough people better to empty whole wards. Nowadays, improvements are less dramatic. Many of the new drugs that have come out recently are really variations on themes established in the 1950's. Usually they are improvements not because they are more effective in making people better, but because they have less in the way of side effects. However, when people carp at the use and possible overuse of medication in psychiatry, it is worth remembering that dramatic beginning.

New drug treatments in psychiatry arise because pharmaceutical companies develop new preparations. These have to undergo very careful testing to establish their effectiveness and freedom from side effects before they are granted a licence and can be prescribed in the normal way.

Most people will be offered some sort of medication during their hospital admission and during home treatment. Although medication is never the complete answer to a mental health problem, it is often a necessary first step, providing a platform on which other types of treatment can build. In the treatment of psychiatric conditions, medication is often continued after a person returns home, sometimes for many months or years. Many people have expressed worries that psychiatrists use these drugs merely in order to keep patients quiet, and that large doses are prescribed without proper consideration of their possible bad effects. There were real grounds for this worry, but most psychiatrists these days weigh the benefits and disadvantages of treatment very carefully. Nevertheless, if you feel that you see changes in your relatives that might be due to the unwanted effects of medication, it is reasonable to share your worry with the psychiatrist in charge of treatment. However, such changes can be the result, not only of the drugs, but of the underlying condition, so it is difficult to be sure of their cause. This section will describe the sorts of effects that may arise from taking the medication that psychiatrists commonly use.

One of the problems with medication in this country is that all medical drugs have at least two names. This can be confusing. First is the approved or 'generic' name of the compound – examples include diazepam or imipramine. Then the pharmaceutical companies give their product their own name, which is different – so diazepam may become Valium, and imipramine Tofranil. The company name is distinguished from the generic name by having a capital initial letter. If, as sometimes happens, several companies each have their own brand of a drug, the picture becomes very complicated indeed. Doctors are encouraged to use the generic names, but they often don't. In this book, we use the generic name, sometimes with most common pharmaceutical name in brackets.

There are several different sorts of medication that may be prescribed for the severe mental illnesses we are concerned with here. They can be given in tablet or capsule form, as a sort of syrup, or, in an emergency, by injection. Some drugs are available in a long acting formulation, and they are given by injection weekly or less frequently. Many people end up preferring this long-acting medication, as it doesn't have to be taken so often and they don't have to worry about remembering when tablets are due. It does mean that some of the control of medication is taken from the patient, as the drug remains in the body for a few weeks after the last injection. Some find this unacceptable.

The medicine given to patients will vary according to the type of illness they have. Schizophrenia is usually treated with a group of drugs variously termed *major tranquillizers*, *antipsychotics* or *neuroleptics* (these terms all refer to the same type of drug). Examples you might have heard of include chlorpromazine (Largactil), haloperidol (Serenace) or fluphenazine decanoate (Modecate), but there are now many of these drugs available. We list them in Tables 1, 2 and 3. Acute attacks of mania are also usually treated with medicines from this group.

TABLE 1
'CONVENTIONAL' MAJOR TRANQUILLIZERS

Name	Proprietary name	Common Side-effects
chlorpromazine	Largactil	Blurred vision,
flupentixol	Depixol	Constipation, difficulty in
fluphenazine	Moditen	passing water, dry mouth,
haloperidol	Haldol, Serenace, Dozic	faintness on suddenly
levopromazine	Nozinan	standing up,
pericyazine	Neulactil	increased appetite.
perphenazine	Fentazin	Loss of facial expression,
pimozide	Orap	odd movements of the body
sulpiride	Dolmatil, Sulpor, Sulpitil	and face, restlessness,
thioridazine	Melleril[1]	stiffness, tremor.
trifluoperazine	Stelazine	Sensitivity of skin to sunlight.
zuclopenthixol	Clopixol	Lowering of body temperature.
		Increased effect of alcohol.

Not every drug shows all of these effects to the same extent. Side-effects are often temporary.

1 The Committee on Safety of Medicines states this should only be used as a second line treatment of schizophrenia and only under the supervision of a mental health specialist because of its effects on the heart.

TABLE 2
NEW ('ATYPICAL') MAJOR TRANQUILLISERS

Name	Proprietary Name	Side-effects
clozapine	Clozaril	Does not produce shaking, stiffness or abnormal movements. Sometimes works where other drugs fail. Can cause a dangerous drop in white blood cells. Needs monitoring with a regular blood test. Other side-effects include drowsiness, drooling, weight gain and epileptic fits.
sertindole	Serdolect	Only rarely produces shaking stiffness or abnormal movements. Can be taken once daily. Can produce dry mouth, blurred vision, dizziness and weight gain. Was withdrawn because of effects on heart rhythm, and has been reintroduced for use only under very restricted conditions.
risperidone	Risperdal	Relatively rarely produces shaking, stiffness or abnormal movements. Can be taken once daily. Makes some people anxious, others sleepy. Relatively little weight gain. Stomach upsets. Dizziness.
olanzapine	Zyprexa	Only rarely produces shaking, stiffness or abnormal movements. Can be taken once daily. Sleepiness, weight gain, dry mouth, blurred vision and dizziness. The major problem with this drug in clinical practice is its tendency to cause weight gain. There is increasing evidence that olanzapine causes diabetes
quetiapine	Seroquel	Little tendency to produce movement disorders, sexual side-effects or serious blood disorders. Mildly sedating, causing drowsiness in some people. May not control psychotic symptoms as well as other drugs from this group.
zotepine	Zoleptil	Minor tendencies only towards weight gain, drowsiness, dry mouth, akathisia, low blood pressure, rapid heartbeat constipation, indigestion.

Table 2 Continued

Name	Proprietary Name	Side-effects
aripiprazole	Abilify	Good side-effect profile. Few neuromuscular side-effects. Very new.

These probably represent an advance on earlier drugs, but they do have their own drawbacks, particularly clozapine and sertindole. The NICE recommendations are discussed on page 108. Atypical antipsychotics may affect driving and other skilled tasks. The effects of alcohol are enhanced.They are all very expensive, but one would probably want one's own relative to have a drug from this group.

The major tranquillizers are so called because of their effects on severe psychiatric disturbance. The minor tranquillizers, such as diazepam (Valium), work in a different way and are used for different conditions, although they are now sometimes used to treat the agitation often associated with psychosis. The major tranquillizers do tranquillize, that is, they calm people down, but their particular effect is to reduce the more disturbing symptoms, such as hallucinations, odd ideas or difficulties in thinking. In most people this means the more severe problems of the illness can be controlled, but it may not mean they disappear completely, and the drugs may not be effective all the time. While the major tranquillizers are often very effective in treating the more dramatic features of the illness they have little effect on negative symptoms. Unlike the minor tranquillizers, the major tranquillizers do not seem to be addictive.

These drugs do not necessarily make someone with schizophrenia or mania *feel* better, even when their benefits are obvious to others. During a straightforward physical illness like an infection, it is usually quickly obvious that medication reduces fever and improves wellbeing. In contrast, drugs used for these severe mental illnesses may have no effects discernible to the person taking them, who may even feel worse for a time. Sometimes this is due to the fact it may take some days or weeks before the benefits of major tranquillizers become apparent. It is not quite clear why the drugs have this delayed effect, as the proper levels of the drug in the body are reached quite quickly. However, for someone who does not agree that there is anything wrong with them, being given drugs that seem unnecessary can be very disturbing.

You yourself may also find this issue very difficult, if you too are unable to see immediate benefits of drug treatment. However, carers are usually only too well aware that their relative's refusal to take their medication has a bad effect on the course of their illness. Their help in encouraging patients to take their drugs can be crucial. The medication can then work to help patients become gradually more in touch with reality and easier to talk to.

Most medicines have several effects: the unwanted ones are called side-effects. Perhaps the most obvious are the neuromuscular movement disorders which can result from taking them. Because of the particular brain connections that underlie the side effects, these symptoms are called extrapyramidal. There are a number of different types of movement disorder associated with anntipsychotic drugs. They include parkinsonism, akinesia, akathisia, dystonia, dysphonia and oculogyric crisis. The first of these involves symptoms rather like those of Parkinson's disease – slowing, restlessness, trembling and muscle stiffness. Sufferers may find it difficult to move, and their muscles may feel stiff and weak. This in turn can result in a loss of facial animation. The condition may affect the way people walk, so they lean forward taking small steps. They may find it difficult to start and stop walking. Finally sufferers often shake, particularly in their hands. This so-called 'drug-induced Parkinsonism' usually passes off in a few weeks, and in any case it is possible to treat it with the drugs that are usually used in Parkinson's disease. However, these days, psychiatrists feel that side-effects of this type indicate that the drug is being used in too high a dose.

Akathisia is a drug-induced restlessness. Patients may feel so restless they are unable to sit still, and they may often feel emotionally very tense as well. The urge to move is often overwhelming, and patients have particular difficulty in keeping their legs still. Once more it can be treated by prescribing additional drugs, although it is again better if the dose of medication is chosen so that this side-effect does not appear in the first place.

Another neuromuscular side-effect of antipsychotic medication involves muscle spasms (dystonia, dysphonia and oculogyric crisis). Muscles suddenly contract uncontrollably. This can be painful, as you might imagine. The contractions often affect the limbs, but when they affect the muscles of the larynx, as they sometimes do, it makes it difficult to speak normally (dysphonia). Sometimes the muscles that control eye movements are affected. The usual result of this is that the eyes turn suddenly upwards in an uncontrollable manner (an oculogyric crisis). This is very unpleasant, and potentially dangerous, and it looks very strange indeed to onlookers.

The final neuromuscular side-effect is 'tardive dyskinesia', over which there is particular concern. This movement disorder is not immediate, but comes on after many months or years of treatment with major tranquillisers. The most prominent and frequent effect is a continual grimacing, which the poor sufferer usually seems unaware of. However the problem can also affect other parts of the body, with muscle spasms, tremors and writhing movements of the limbs. Treatments for this condition have generally been ineffective, and it doesn't normally get better. However, some people are helped by switching to a tranquilliser called clozapine (Table 2), which operates in a slightly different way from the other major tranquillisers. It is not absolutely clear that it is just a drug side effect. Such grimacings were described in schizophrenia long before major tranquillizers, and are still sometimes reported in those who have not yet been prescribed these drugs.

One of the most dangerous side-effects of antipsychotic medication is the neuroleptic malignant syndrome (NMS). It is fortunately rare, occurring in perhaps 1% of hospital patients who take antipsychotic drugs. It usually happens in people under 40 and is commoner in men. People who develop NMS have usually been taking antipsychotic drugs for many years, although not necessarily in very high doses. It often seems to happen soon after the dose of medication has been changed. It develops rapidly (over one to three days), and the first symptoms to appear are usually sweating, rigidity and a high temperature. Other symptoms include tremor, difficulty speaking and swallowing, and changes in consciousness ranging from lethargy and confusion to coma. The heartbeat is rapid, as is breathing, and there are changes in blood pressure. The first line of treatment is to control the fever, and drugs may be given to relax the muscles and to counteract the chemical imbalance that is thought to cause NMS. The condition is dangerous. Up to one in 10 of people getting it may die. Moreover, people who have had it on one occasion are at increased risk of getting it again, and their medication requires to be handled very carefully. Like many of the side-effects of antipsychotic medication, the condition was described in people with psychosis long before the medication was available. When it happens in people who are not on medication, the mechanisms are probably similar to those involved in the type associated with antipsychotics.

The antipsychotic drugs also have effects on sexual function. This is because they increase the level of the hormonal prolactin in the blood. It is only relatively recently that psychiatrists have become fully aware of the extent of these problems. This is because psychiatrists have not tended to raise the issue of sexual function with their severely mentally ill patients, possibly thinking it better to leave well alone. Their patients have been equally reticent. Unfortunately, they frequently responded to these side-effects by quietly and not unreasonably stopping their medication.

The sexual side-effects of antipsychotic drugs can be very noticeable. Both men and women may experience breast development and the production of milk. Sexual desire can be adversely affected in both sexes. This may reduce arousal, and it can cause impotence and sterility in men. Some drugs interfere with erection and ejaculation. Women may experience loss of periods, vaginal dryness, acne and unwanted hair. Hormonal changes may also cause osteoporosis in both men and women.

In addition to their action on dopamine, antipsychotic drugs also to a varying extent influence another neurotransmitter substance, acetylcholine. Their effects on this can cause drowsiness, dry mouth, blurred vision, dizziness, constipation, nausea, difficulty in passing water, and sometimes rapid heartbeat. These anticholinergic effects also increase the likelihood of narrow angle glaucoma. In older people, low blood pressure may be a problem, particularly as it makes falls more likely. Coupled with the effect on osteoporosis, this is probably responsible for the relatively high frequency of fractures among people living in hostels.

It took some time to realise that antipsychotic medication is sometimes associated with sudden death. This is particularly likely when high doses are used and more than one type of antipsychotic has been prescribed at the same time. It probably operates through an effect on heart rhythm, and there have been worries that some of the newer antipsychotics have such an effect. Good practice now suggests that people taking antipsychotics should have ECG examinations from time to time. Grapefruit juice is thought to combine with antipsychotics to increase the effect on heart rhythm, and should be avoided by people on antipsychotic medication.

It was long recognised that people with severe psychiatric disorders had a tendency to put on weight, sometimes rather a lot of weight. Unfortunately, this tended to trouble sufferers more than the psychiatrists treating them. It is only recently that there has been a proper appreciation on the part of clinicians of the scale of this problem. At one time it was regarded as an inevitable consequence of inactivity, and only to be expected. It is now clear that much of the weight gain is due to the effect of antipsychotic medication on appetite, and on the way the body uses food and stores it as fat. This applies to several of the newer drugs, as to some of the older ones. There may be severe health consequences, in particular heart problems and diabetes. Clearly people who already suffer from these diseases, or who have a family history of them, are particularly at risk.

There are a number of other side-effects including blood disorders, liver disorders, skin problems, and difficulties in regulating body temperature. Elderly people taking these drugs may be at particular risk of becoming too cold or too hot in extreme weather.

Because of their tendency towards particular types of side-effects, it is perhaps not surprising that antipsychotics must be used with caution in people with pre-existing medical conditions of various types. These include liver and kidney disorders, heart disease, Parkinson's disease, epilepsy, myasthenia gravis, and prostate enlargement. People who already have a personal or family history of the condition are at increased risk of of angle-closure glaucoma. Caution is also required in severe lung disease and in people with a history of jaundice or blood disorders. Antipsychotics should be used with caution in the elderly, who are particularly susceptible to fainting due to low blood pressure, particularly if they stand up suddenly.

Given this litany of side effects that may result from taking antipsychotic medication, it is perhaps something of a wonder that anybody benefits from taking them. However, for most patients, an optimum balance can be achieved between the untoward effects and the beneficial calming effects of the tranquillizing drugs. However, those who are not convinced of the benefits can become very concerned with the side effects, and may refuse to take any medication at all. Unfortunately, this sometimes means the initial illness returns. In the same way that they take some time to build up a therapeutic effect, the drugs often take some days or weeks to wear off. This means there may be no immediate change when patients stop taking them, so they may feel their decision was justified.

David was a man of 22 who was admitted to hospital because he was acutely disturbed. He had been rushing out of his house, shouting at passers-by and telling them to leave him alone. He thought they were spying on him and that there was an evil and complicated plot afoot to harm him. He continued to be upset in hospital and he was given chlorpromazine, at first in moderate doses, but when this did not have any effect, in quite large doses. Over a period of a few days he settled down and was less frightened. Gradually he lost his delusional ideas and was able to take part in the ward activities. He did become quite shaky for about ten days, almost certainly as a result of the chlorpromazine. However, this wore off without the need either for reducing the dose or for giving further medication to neutralise it. After about eight weeks he was discharged but it was felt that he should continue to take medication, although in much lower doses. In fact he still takes it, and it seems to have been effective in preventing the return of his frightening persecutory ideas. He did discontinue it for a few weeks, but was strongly advised to start it again when he had a minor return of his old suspiciousness.

David's experience with medication was a happy one, and he had no objection to continuing with it. He did not like to talk about the ideas he had, and gave the impression this was because he thought they showed him in rather a foolish light. It appeared though that he thought of medication as a small price to pay to prevent their return. This story was included in the first edition of this book, and these days psychiatrists are particularly careful about using doses of antipsychotic medication that do not cause side effects.

Clearly not all individuals are equally happy with medication. In some this will be because they think they never needed it or at any rate no longer need it, in others because they have side effects they don't like. In some very severe cases of schizophrenia, the psychiatrist may prescribe medication with the hope of only marginal benefit. This can be a very fine judgement, and psychiatrists have a tendency to err on the cautious side, being reluctant to take the risk of discontinuing someone's medication

even when it does not appear to be having any benefit. The problem
is they can never be quite sure that things will not get worse if they
do take their patient off medication. These days they are becoming
more wary of the possibility of doing harm with major
tranquillizers. Under these circumstances of having to weigh the
balance of advantage so carefully, it might happen that you see
things differently from your relative's psychiatrist. This may be
because either you or they do not have all the information against
which the correct prescription of medication must be judged. If you
feel strongly about this, talking to your relative's psychiatrist will at
least clear the air, and may lead to a modification of treatment.

It is in fact possible for some people with schizophrenia even of
a fairly enduring type to manage without medication, although this
is sometimes at the cost of a more restricted life style by which they
avoid overstimulation. Provided they are not actually a danger to
themselves or to others, this is a choice they have a right to make,
although it may make things harder for those who look after them,
whether relatives or clinicians.

Since we wrote the first edition of the book in 1987 there have been
advances in the drug treatment of schizophrenia, and you may have
heard of some of these (see Table 2). Most of these advances concern
the so-called *atypical antipsychotics*. These are supposed to work by
slightly different mechanisms from the older *typical or conventional
antipsychotics* like chlorpromazine (Largactil) and haloperidol
(Serenace), although there is probably as much variation between the
atypical antipsychotics as there is between them and the older drugs.
The pharmaceutical companies have been able to sell atypical
antipsychotics despite their considerable expense because they
appear to cause less in the way of side-effects than their older
counterparts. In particular they seem to produce much less in the way
of extrapyramidal side-effects like drug induced parkinsonism.
Extrapyramidal side-effects are the major cause for people
discontinuing their antipsychotic medication. This is because they
are experienced as very unpleasant. It is probably the case that the
newer antipsychotics produce less in the way of side-effects like this,
but some of the apparent advantage over the older drugs probably
arose because the latter were prescribed in doses that were far too
high. If they use the older drugs, most psychiatrists these days
employ much lower doses than used to be the case.

TABLE 3
Equivalent doses of some antipsychotics

Oral antipsychotics	
Preparation	*Daily dose*
Chlorpromazine	100 mg
Clozapine	50 mg
Haloperidol	2–3 mg
Pimozide	2 mg
Risperidone	0.5–1 mg
Sulpiride	200 mg
Thioridazine	100 mg
Trifluoperazine	5 mg

Depot antipsychotics		
Preparation	*Dose (mg)*	*Interval between injections*
Flupentixol decanoate	40	2 weeks
Fluphenazine decanoate	25	2 weeks
Haloperidol decanoate	100	4 weeks
Pipotiazine palmitate	50	4 weeks
Zuclopenthixol decanoate	200	2 weeks

In Britain we now have access to authoritative opinions about medication from the National Institute for Clinical Excellence (NICE). This is part of the NHS. It was set up to evaluate the evidence about treatments for the whole range of medical disorders with a view to producing guidance for health care professionals, patients and carers to help them make decisions about treatments and health care. It was launched in mid-2000. It sifts evidence with great care in order to come to the clearest possible view of how things stand.

The recent NICE guidelines on the treatment of schizophrenia have been very influential. They recommend that doctors use antipsychotics at the lowest effective dose, and introduce the drugs gradually. They particularly emphasise that people should not be given a high starting dose. They say the atypical antipsychotics should be considered for the first-line treatment of newly diagnosed schizophrenia. They should be chosen for managing acute schizophrenic episodes when discussion with the individual is not possible. They should also be considered when someone experiences unacceptable side-effects with a conventional antipsychotic. They should be considered for treating relapse where symptoms were not in any case previously well controlled. However, quite reasonably the guidelines do not suggest changing to an atypical antipsychotic if symptoms are adequately controlled by one of the older antipsychotics and there are no unacceptable side-effects. Finally they recommend changing to clozapine when schizophrenia has been inadequately controlled despite the use of two or more antipsychotics in turn for at least 6–8 weeks each. One of these should have been an atypical antipsychotic.

The effect of the introduction of the new drugs, and the more refined prescription of the older drugs has been quite revolutionary. It is now extremely rare to see people with a severe mental illness who are marked out by their stiffness and shaking. This is clearly of great importance, as looking like that was extremely stigmatising.

SOME ANTIPSYCHOTIC DRUGS

The oldest of the old typical drugs is chlorpromazine (Largactil). In fact it is not very typical at all, having multiple effects. This is the reason for its drug company name, which refers to the large range of actions that it has. It is one of the more sedating drugs, which can be an advantage in some circumstances, particularly in the early phase of the illness which may be characterised by disturbed behaviour. Because of its anticholinergic effects, it can cause blurred vision and low blood pressure. Many people gain quite a lot of weight when they use it. It occasionally causes blood clots and damage the liver. It makes people extra sensitive to sunlight. Despite the fact that it has been around a long time, chlorpromazine remains a useful drug, particularly if used in proper doses. In the past, it was used in doses up to 2000 mg a day. Nowadays this would be regarded as much too high, and most people's illness can be controlled on around 300 mg per day, once they are stabilised. There is evidence that increasing the dose above this confers no additional benefit but causes an increase in side-effects.

Another of the old drugs that remains in common use is haloperidol (Serenace, Haldol). This is less sedating them chlorpromazine and has fewer of the anticholinergic effects.

However it does produce more neuromuscular side-effects, particularly muscle spasms and akathisia. It also sometimes produces effects on the liver and on gastrointestinal function. This is another drug that has in the past been used in rather high doses, up to 30 mg a day. The rate of side-effects increases very considerably in doses above 10 mg a day. For most people, their illness can be controlled at doses of around 6 mg a day. Trifluoperazine (Stelazine) is rather like haloperidol in its side-effect profile. Fluphenazine (Moditen) is another drug in the older group that is still prescribed and, like haloperidol, its side-effects tend to be neuromuscular. Flupentixol (Depixol) is also still used: in its actions it is rather like fluphenazine, although it produces fewer neuromuscular side-effects, and may have some antidepressant activity. Pimozide (Orap) is another of the older antipsychotic drugs. It is less sedating than chlorpromazine; relatively recently it has been associated with serious disturbances in heart rhythm, particularly in higher doses. Sulpiride (Dolmatil) is also less sedating than chlorpromazine. It is not associated with liver damage or skin reactions, and in most people does not cause weight gain. It does have adverse effects on sexual function. Nevertheless this is probably one of the cleanest of the older drugs, particularly if used in moderate doses (well below the recommended maximum limit of 2.4 g per day).

A number of other typical antipsychotic drugs continue to be produced, but are prescribed only rarely.

The atypical antipsychotic drugs are relatively new. Most of them were introduced in the 1990s, and they have always been sold on the basis that they do not produce the neuromuscular side-effects of the older drugs. Some, but not all, have less effect on sexual function than the older drugs. All the members of this group are expensive. In some parts of the country, particularly in the early days of their introduction, psychiatrists have been discouraged from using atypical antipsychotic medication on grounds of cost.

Clozapine (Clozaril) is actually quite an old drug that was originally discontinued because, as we shall see, it had one particularly severe, if fairly rare, side-effect. However it acts somewhat differently from the other drugs in this field. This means it has little in the way of the usual side-effects like shaking and movement disorder. Indeed it can be prescribed as a way of reducing those side-effects. Its great benefit however is that it is effective in a proportion (perhaps as many as 50%) of those people who do not recover much in response to the other drugs. We have seen people very disabled by severe mental illness become much more able to look after themselves as a result of being switched to clozapine.

The big disadvantage of clozapine is that it causes a serious reduction in the number of white cells in the blood in perhaps 1-2% of the people who take it. This means they cannot fight infections properly. A few people have died as a result. For this reason, those who take clozapine have to have blood taken, at first on a weekly basis, then fortnightly, eventually monthly, to make sure their white blood cells are all right. If the level starts to fall beyond a certain point, the clozapine has to be stopped. This side-effect has two consequences in everybody who takes the drug: the blood tests are an inconvenience, and the drug is very expensive because the cost of these tests has to be covered. If patients miss their regular blood tests, the drug company involved prohibit them from receiving the drug. If they are once more persuaded of the need to take the drug and to agree to the blood tests, the treatment has to start again at the beginning. Clozapine can only be given by mouth, not as a long-acting injection. This means people reluctant to take medication anyway may default on taking it, which may also lead the drug company to prohibit its continued prescription. A further unusual side-effect is a tendency to produce too much saliva, particularly at night. People on clozapine may wake to find their pillow drenched. However, this side-effect does wear off and can be reduced by reducing the dose of the drug. Clozapine also causes epilepsy in a small percentage of patients. There is an increasing appreciation that weight gain is very common with this drug, and this may lead to diabetes in some people treated with it.

The pharmaceutical industry is always on the lookout for the 'son of clozapine', that is, a drug with all its advantages of effectiveness and reduced side-effects but with no effect on white cells. It is not clear that any of the new or upcoming drugs fit this description.

Risperidone (Risperdal) was the second atypical antipsychotic drug to be licensed for use. It produces more neuromuscular side-effects than clozapine, but less than the older antipsychotic drugs. When risperidone was first introduced, the manufacturers recommended doses that were almost certainly too high. Their allowable range was from two to 16 mg per day. However if the dose is kept below six or at most 8 mg a day it usually provides good control of the illness, without causing neuromuscular side-effects. It does not affect white blood cells – so no blood test is required. It is usually slightly sedating, although in some people it can be arousing, leading to insomnia, agitation and anxiety. It produces some weight gain but is not as bad as some of the other antipsychotic drugs in this respect. In some people it produces sexual side-effects. It is available as an ordinary tablet, but now there is also a version that can be dissolved under the tongue. It is the only atypical antipsychotic drug that can be prescribed as a long-acting injection.

The next atypical to come on the market was olanzapine (Zyprexa). This drug produces relatively little in the way of acute side-effects, and rarely produces movement disorders. It can produce drowsiness and oedema (puffness of the feet and hands). While in some people it causes changes in blood levels of the sex hormone prolactin, it produces little in the way of sexual side-effects. The major problem with this drug in clinical practice is its tendency to cause weight gain. It is possibly the worst antipsychotic drug in this respect. Some people gain several stones in weight, and they find it hard to control this with diet and exercise. There is sometimes an assumption that people with severe mental illness do not care about their appearance. While in some cases this may be true, there are also many people who are mortified by their obesity. It is a major reason for discontinuing medication. In addition, there is increasing evidence that olanzapine causes diabetes in some people. It may also cause increases in blood fats. Thus although it offers good control of psychotic symptoms without movement disorders, it must be used carefully if it is not to contribute to the very poor physical health endured by many people with severe mental illnesses.

Quetiapine (Seroquel) is another of the atypical antipsychotic drugs. It has little tendency to produce movement disorders and this is one of its major advantages. It does not raise prolactin levels and therefore does not produce sexual side-effects. Nor is there an association with serious blood disorders. It is mildly sedating and therefore causes drowsiness in some people. It sometimes reduces an increased heart rate. Psychiatrists regard it as a 'clean' drug, but one that is sometimes less effective in controlling psychotic symptoms than other drugs from this group.

Amisulpride (Solian) is closely related to sulpiride, and has a very similar mode of action and side-effect profile. Despite this, it is included among the atypical antipsychotics, while its brother is regarded as typical. It is not surprising therefore that it offers good control of psychotic symptoms, is relatively free of neuromuscular side-effects, and is prone to produce sexual problems.

Sertindole (Serdolect) was withdrawn by the makers after reports of serious effects on heart rhythm that might have been linked to sudden death. After further investigation it has been reintroduced, but only on a 'named patient' basis. It is restricted to people who are involved in clinical studies and to those who have responded badly to at least one other antipsychotic. People starting as drug need to be screened first with an electrocardiogram (ECG). Part of the problem for pharmaceutical companies who introduce new drugs is that, very properly, these are placed under close surveillance. The principle is that potentially dangerous side-effects are picked up at an early stage. The older drugs were not so subject to this rigorous surveillance, and we are becoming aware that effects on heart rate and heart rhythm are more common than was thought in most of the antipsychotic drugs (for instance, with thioridazine). It is beginning to look like good routine clinical practice to give people ECGs before starting long-term treatment with antipsychotic medication.

Zotepine (Zoleptil) is relatively new. It has many of the side-effects that are seen with antipsychotic medication in general(weight gain, drowsiness, dry mouth, akathisia, low blood pressure, rapid heartbeat, constipation, indigestion for instance), but these are usually relatively mild, and relatively infrequent. While it does produce sexual side-effects, these are not usually a problem at lower doses.

Aripiprazole (Abilify) is the newest of the atypical antipsychotics, having been introduced in mid-2004. It seems to be effective and to have a good side-effect profile. In particular, it produces little in the way of neuromuscular side-effects. Like any new drug, it will be some time before we have a clear view of its advantages and disadvantages.

LONG ACTING ANTIPSYCHOTIC DRUGS (DEPOT INJECTIONS)

As indicated above, some antipsychotic drugs can be given as a 'slow-release' preparation. These are given by deep injection into a muscle, sometimes the shoulder muscle, but usually into the gluteus maximus, which is the large muscle of the bottom. Some people find this rather undignified. These days the injections are often given by a community psychiatric nurse who will visit their clients at home to do this. Because the drugs are long acting they can be given at intervals usually of between one week and one month. Long acting preparations based on the drugs flupentixol, fluphenazine, and haloperidol have been around for many years. At one time they were given over long periods without proper review, and the dosages used were often rather high, particularly as each of these drugs causes neuromuscular reactions. In addition to the general side-effects of antipsychotic medication, the drug is dissolved in a sort of oil, and this can cause pain in the muscle at the site of the injection. Moreover, the oil is obtained from various nuts, and people with nut allergies should avoid these preparations. Thus flupentixol decanoate (Depixol) is suspended in coconut oil, while fluphenazine decanoate (Modecate), haloperidol decanoate (Haldol) and pipothiazine palmitate (Piportil) use sesame oil. Of these drugs flupentixol and pipothiazine cause least in the way of neuromuscular side-effects. Flupentixol may have some antidepressant properties which are sometimes useful in their own right.

The only atypical antipsychotic available so far in a long acting form is risperidone (Risperdal Consta). It is best used for people who have already been successfully treated with risperidone tablets, at least at some stage even if not recently, and who now want to receive their medication by injection. The formulation is not oil-based. The drug is supplied as a powder and a solvent. This is made up at the time of injection, as it has a very short shelf-life. The side-effects are those of risperidone in tablet form, and because the injection is not oil-based, persistent pain at the site of injection does not occur.

In principle, this formulation should represent a treatment advance. There is a problem however. Following the first injection, the drug takes a few weeks before adequate blood levels are achieved. When the injection regime is first started, this usually makes for a rather difficult balancing act, whereby the oral risperidone dose is reduced as the drug from the injection comes on stream. Likewise, once the injection regime is established, juggling with the dose is very much in slow motion. The effect of dose modifications cannot be seen for some weeks. If it is given to somebody whose mental state varies more quickly than this, the room for error is increased. This formulation is therefore best for people who are fairly stable anyway. Moreover the experience of some psychiatrists is that in the recommended doses, the preparation is less effective than risperidone by mouth. This formulation is still new, and it is likely to be some time before people become fully experienced in using it, and before its place in treatment options is clear.

TREATING DEPRESSION WITH MEDICATION

Depressed mood, whether part of a severe depressive illness, schizo-affective disorder or schizophrenia, is usually treated with antidepressants. These are all believed to operate by restoring the chemical imbalance that probably underlies moderate and severe depression, that is, by an effect on neurotransmitters. They increase the level of particular neurotransmitters, especially noradrenaline and serotonin. They have the aim of prolonging the effects of the neurotransmitters either by stopping them being taken back up into the cell they were released by or by stopping them being broken down by enzymes.

There are three main groups. Over the last fifty years the most commonly used group has been the tricyclic antidepressants. This includes drugs like imipramine, amitriptyline, dothiepin and maprotiline (see Table 4). Again, there are many for the doctor to choose from. Tricyclic antidepressants are so called because their chemical structure takes the form of three linked rings. They affect both noradrenaline and serotonin, although predominantly the former. Some non-tricyclic drugs have a similar chemical structure and action (maprotiline, mianserin and trazadone). The tricyclic drugs have a rather broad chemical action, and affect other transmitter systems as well. These are responsible for some of side-effects. The anticholinergic effects cause drowsiness dry mouth, blurred vision, constipation, rapid heartbeat, difficulty in passing water, and sweating. The effects on the heart are particularly dangerous in overdose. Because tricyclic antidepressants can cause drowsiness, they affect people's ability to perform particular tasks such as driving or operating machinery. Elderly people are particularly prone to the side-effects.

Another group of drugs, which go by the catchy name of selective serotonin reuptake inhibitors (SSRIs), were developed after the first edition of this book. In the 1990s, they were increasingly chosen because they have much less in the way of side-effects than the tricyclic antidepressants. They were responsible for raising the awareness of doctors and patients alike about the possibility of treating depression effectively, and as a result more people with depressive disorders are prescribed these drugs by their family doctors. The most famous of these to the general public is Prozac (fluoxetine). Because they are relatively new, they are however usually expensive, although two of them are now out of their license period and have come down in price. There are also drugs which combined the ability to inhibit the reuptake of serotonin and of noradrenaline. The best known is venlafaxine, which at one point looked as though it was more effective than the other antidepressant drugs. However there are now grave doubts about its safety.

The final group, the monoamine oxidase inhibitors (MAOI's), includes phenelzine and tranyleypramine but is used less often (Table 4). However, there is a relatively new 'reversible' MAOI (moclobamide), which is likely to be a useful addition to the list of antidepressants.

Some antidepressants are very dangerous indeed in overdose. They may cause convulsions and have direct effect on the heart which leads to death if enough of the drug has been taken.

Although antidepressants are absorbed quickly into the body, they take to between two and four weeks to be effective (we do not know why this is so). It takes a few days before mood even starts to lift, so the tablets have to be taken exactly as prescribed. It is likely to be several weeks, and in some cases even longer, before mood is completely normal, and the psychiatrist will probably continue to prescribe this medication for some time after that.

Antidepressants do have some immediate effects. Some make patients feel drowsy, others may have an energising effect. This may interfere with the patient's ability to drive. Complaints of a dry mouth or of blurred vision are fairly common, but these side effects usually become less noticeable over a few days. The effects of alcohol are increased in people taking these drugs. The SSRI's only rarely have these side-effects although they have some of their own: they can increase anxiety for a few days and they can make some people feel quite nauseated. Nevertheless, they are usually more acceptable than the older tricyclic antidepressants. The MAOI

TABLE 4
Antidepressants

Tricyclic antidepressants	Drug company name	Common side effects
Amoxapine	Asendis	Dry mouth, blurred vision,
Clomipramine	Anafranil	constipation, difficulty in passing
	Dosulepin (dothiepin)	water, weight gain, confusion in the elderly.
	Prothiaden	Increased effect of alcohol.
	Doxepin	Occasional worsening of
	Sinequan	of symptoms in those
Imipramine	Tofranil	with schizophrenia.
Lofepramine	Gamamil, Lomont	*Side-effects tend to wear off over a few*
Maprotiline	Ludiomil	*days and are less*
	Nortriptyline	*prominent if the dose*
	Allegron	*is gradually increased*
Trimipramine	Surmontil	*to full levels.*

SSRIs		
Citalopram	Cipramil	Nausea, diarrhoea, headache, insomnia,
Escitalopram	Cipralex	agitation, and sexual dysfunction.
Fluoxetine	Prozac	Less dry mouth , blurred vision,
Fluvoxamine	Faverin	constipation, or difficulty in passing
Paroxetine	Seroxat	water than tricyclic antidepressants.
Sertraline	Lustral	Safer in overdose.

MAOIs		
Isocarboxazid		Interaction with foods (see table), with
Moclobemide	Manerix	alcohol and other prescribed drugs.
(Reversible)		Interactions with moclobemide are less.
Phenelzine	Nardil	Faintness on standing.
Tranylcypromine	Parnate	

Other types		
Mirtazapine	Zispin	Specific to the drugs.
Reboxetine	Edronax	
Trazodone	Molipaxin	
Venlafaxine	Efexor	

In addition, the antipsychotic flupentixol is sometimes used (in low doses) because it has some antidepressant effect.

TABLE 5
Foods to be avoided by those taking Monoamine Oxidase Inhibitors

Cheese (especially cream cheese)
Meat and yeast extracts (eg. Bovril, Marmite, Oxo)
Broad Beans
Avocado pears
Pickled herrings
Food which might be 'going off' (especially meat, fish, poultry)
Proprietary cough and cold medicines (i.e. bought over the counter at a pharmacists)
Chocolate, yoghurt, cream and game may also produce reactions, although more rarely.
The effect of alcohol is increased by these drugs, but in addition red wine can set off the same reaction as the foods above.

group of antidepressants interact with certain foodstuffs that contain high levels of tyramine, particularly cheese. These reactions can be dangerous: there is a rapid rise in blood pressure with severe headache. Very occasionally, the reaction can trigger off a stroke. Patients prescribed this type of drug are given cards by the pharmacy listing all the foods to be avoided. This list is given in Table 5. The newest drug from this group, moclobamide, very rarely interacts with tyramine, so no dietary restrictions are needed. It has very few other side-effects. However, before switching to moclobamide it is necessary to wait until the blood is cleared of previously prescribed antidepressants (a 'washout' period).

You will remember Sue, the depressed teacher we spoke of in Chapter One. You might like to know what happened to her. She was suffering from the sort of depression that a psychiatrist would immediately recognise as likely to benefit from an antidepressant. She was prescribed dothiepin (Prothiaden – which we would not choose these days because it is particularly dangerous in overdose), although she would probably have responded equally to any of the other antidepressants. At first she was given a small dose, but over a few days this was increased to a moderately large one. This gradual introduction of the drug was deliberate, as it lessens the chance of side-effects. She did notice her mouth was dry, and she felt a little bit unsteady and sleepy. In fact she was feeling pretty rotten anyway, so the sleepiness did not matter and, if anything, took the edge off her anguish. At first, there was little change, but after a fortnight or so she was able to report a slight lightening in the gloom. Over the following few weeks she gradually improved, and after two months was able to return to work. She had started enjoying herself again. Her husband was delighted to have back the wife he had known. She was once more a sociable, loving and energetic woman. Apart from the antidepressant, little treatment was required beyond support through the bad period, and some advice about the general management of her life. The medication was continued for about three months after she had fully recovered. Just occasionally, someone who appears completely better may relapse if antidepressants are stopped too quickly.

In December 2004, NICE published its guidelines for the treatment of depression. These are quite interesting, in that the very careful and clear interpretation of the evidence from research pointed the way to unexpected conclusions. The underlying principle is that the management of depression should be based on something called 'stepped care'. The guidelines emphasise the need for family doctors and doctors in general hospitals to screen people for depression. However, for those with mild depression, they recommended that health care professionals should not actually provide treatment, but keep an eye on the patient ('watchful waiting'). This is because many people with mild depression get better without treatment. Indeed the guidelines do not recommend the use of antidepressants in mild depression. They suggested instead a guided self-help programme based on cognitive behavioural therapy in both mild and moderate depression. If an antidepressant is to be used, they recommend that it should be a selective serotonin reuptake inhibitor (SSRI), as the evidence has shown that these are as effective as tricyclic antidepressants and less likely to be stopped by the patient because of side-effects.

The guidelines also point out that people may get symptoms if they stop the drug, particularly if they do so suddenly. They recommended that people with a severe depression should be treated if possible with a combination of antidepressants and individual cognitive behaviour therapy. This combination is also recommended for treatment resistant depression.

People with recurrent depression, that is, those who have had at least two moderately severe depressive episodes fairly recently, should receive long-term treatment with antidepressants. If they experience recurrences despite this, CBT is recommended. Again NICE recommends an SSRI in this situation, and states that fluoxetine and citalopram are generally associated with fewest discontinuation or withdrawal symptoms, although fluoxetine has a higher tendency to interact adversely with other drugs. Some treatments, particularly those involving a combination of drugs, should only be carried out by a specialist mental health care professional. Combinations of SSRI antidepressants may result in the 'serotonin syndrome', whereby people experience confusion, delirium, shivering, sweating, changes in blood pressure, and myoclonus.

The NICE guidelines are particularly wary of the drug venlafaxine, and indicate that this too should only be managed by specialist mental health clinicians. Venlafaxine is particularly likely to lead to people dropping out of treatment because of side-effects. If patients do discontinue it suddenly, it has a strong tendency to cause discontinuation and withdrawal symptoms. It is also toxic in overdose. Blood pressure needs to be monitored, and patients may need electrocardiographs (ECGs) from time to time.

One of the considerations underlying the guidelines is that when these drugs are taken in overdose, the tricyclic antidepressants (apart from lofepramine) are more dangerous.

Antidepressants should be discontinued gradually. Patients who stop their antidepressant suddenly, and even those who miss a dose or just reduce their dosage, may experience discontinuation and withdrawal symptoms. It is reasonable to reduce dosage gradually over a four-week period.

If someone does not response to the first antidepressant prescribed, the advice is to change to another antidepressant after a month or so. The choice of a second antidepressant includes a different SSRI, mirtazepine, moclobemide, reboxetine and tricyclic antidepressants. There are sometimes problems with interactions between antidepressants so the changeover needs to be managed carefully. Mirtazepine can cause sedation and weight gain. Lofepramine is probably the best tricyclic antidepressant to prescribe because it has relatively little in the way of a toxic effect on the heart.

In some people whose depression has failed to respond to several antidepressants it is reasonable to add lithium (see below) to the antidepressant treatment. Before this is done an ECG should be carried out.

There is a certain amount of evidence that the herb St John's wort is helpful for mild or moderate depression. There are problems in taking it, one of which is that the preparations vary in strength and there is no system for standardising them. Moreover it seems to interact badly with SSRI antidepressants.

There has been a lot of comment recently about problems connected with stopping antidepressants. Antidepressants do not usually produce a 'high' and in consequence are not truly addictive. However, to a varying extent, they do cause discontinuation symptoms which include stomach upsets, loss of appetite, various sorts of sleep disturbance, rapid mood changes, and restlessness. Withdrawal from SSRIs in particular may cause dizziness, numbness and sensations like electric shocks.

Patients who have repeated episodes of depression, and especially those who also have experienced an episode of mania, may be prescribed lithium. Whilst this does have an effect on acute symptoms, its main use is to make relapse less likely. It may take a year, or even more, before it can be seen to be effective, and it therefore involves patients taking medication whilst free of symptoms. From time to time the psychiatrist will want a blood test to determine the level of this drug in the body. This is to ensure the correct dose and an absence of side effects, as the correct dose lies in a fairly narrow band between one that is ineffective and one that produces unwanted effects. Monitoring ensures that only a tiny minority of patients suffer significant side-effects. Nevertheless, it can sometimes happen that the level becomes too high. Symptoms that suggest this possibility are listed in Table 6.

TABLE 6
Side effects of lithium

		Action
Early and fleeting	Nausea Diarrhoea Metallic taste	Mention to doctor. Not dangerous
Persistent	Weight gain	Mention to doctor
	Shakiness Increased consumption of water Increased amounts of urine	Mention to doctor as a matter of urgency. It may be necessary to reduce the dose.

Jeremy, a quiet scholarly man who worked in a bank, had experienced three rather damaging breakdowns. The first looked like schizophrenia but by the time of the third it became clear that the likely diagnosis was bipolar disorder. His employers had been tolerant of his problems, despite the fact that his behaviour during episodes had brought adverse publicity to them. However, their tolerance could not be boundless. It was decided to start treatment with lithium, and Jeremy has now taken it for ten years without any recurrence. His only complaint is that he finds it hard to lose weight.

Gillian also did well on lithium. However, she developed considerable swelling of the ankles, and it was decided to take her off the medication. While this was sensible in terms of her physical condition, it did mean she had a return of symptoms from time to time that led to her admission to hospital on two occasions and caused considerable strain for her family.

Recently, it has been found that the drug carbamezepine can be used successfully to prevent the return of bipolar disorder, sometimes in people for whom other treatments have failed. Gillian was started on carbamezepine and has been well ever since. A number of other drugs are now sometimes used to help in mood stabilization, of which the most common is sodium valproate. The evidence for the effectiveness of these other drugs is still rather thin, although they do sometimes seem to work well.

Sometimes if a person suffers from depressive delusions, the psychiatrist will prescribe major tranquillizers like those used in schizophrenia. These can be quite effective in this condition, too. Occasionally, people with these illnesses may be given minor tranquillizers, such as diazepam or lorazepam (see Table 7). These do not help to cure an attack directly, but may calm someone who is particularly agitated. They may be used during acute episodes, or to calm someone very distressed when first admitted to hospital/home treatment. Psychiatrists are increasingly reluctant to prescribe these drugs and will do so only in certain restricted circumstances, as they are now known to be addictive. When they are prescribed, the psychiatrist will these days aim to discontinue them as soon as possible, certainly within a few months, usually within a few weeks. In some cases when people have been taking minor tranquillizers for years, it may be impracticable to discontinue them, especially if other problems seem more important. People aiming to come off these medications after a long period should do so under medical

TABLE 7
Minor tranquillisers and hypnotics

Name	Proprietary name	Common side effects
Benzodiazepines		
Minor tranquillisers		
alprazolam	Xanax	Drowsiness, confusion, impaired performance on physical tasks like driving and operating machinery. Increases the effects of alcohol. Addiction.
chlordiazepoxide	Librium	
clorazepate	Tranxene	
diazepam	Valium	
lorazepam	Ativan	
oxazepam		
Hypnotics		
flurazepam	Dalmane	
loprazolam		
lormetazepam		
nitrazepam	Mogadon	
temazepam	Normison	
clobazepam	Frisium	

Flurazepam and nitrazepam are longer acting than the other three in this group and are therefore more likely to produce a hangover.

Other hypnotics		
zaleplon	Sonata	
zolpidem	Zimovane	
zopiclone	Stilnoct	

These are relatively new. They are not benzodiazepines, but act on benzodiazepine receptors. Dependence has occasionally been reported. Zaleplon, which is particularly short-acting should be prescribed for only 2 weeks, the others for up to 4. Side effects include stomach upset, dizziness, headache.

Other tranquilliser		
buspirone	Buspar	Dizziness, headache, nausea; potential for dependence and abuse seems low

supervision, as there may be withdrawal effects, especially if it is done too quickly. A list of the withdrawal effects is given in Table 8. Some of this group cannot now be prescribed under the NHS.

TABLE 8
Withdrawal symptoms of minor tranquillizers

Apprehension and anxiety
Loss of appetite
Faintness, light headedness or unsteadiness
Fatigue
Sleep disturbance
Shakiness, muscle twitches, muscle cramps in legs.
Pins and needles
Hypersensitivity to sensation
Vomiting.

These symptoms are likely to come on a few days after stopping the medication, and usually do so only after someone has been taking appreciable doses for six months or so. In some instances, the symptoms may appear like 'flu' or gastro-enteritis. They can also resemble an anxiety state, except for the muscle twitches.

ELECTROCONVULSIVE THERAPY (ECT)

The NICE guidelines recommend that ECT is only used to achieve rapid and short-term improvement of severe symptoms after there has been an adequate attempt to treat a patient with other treatments that have proved ineffective. The decision to use ECT should be made jointly by the individual and the clinicians responsible for treatment on the basis of an informed discussion. The course of ECT and its effects should be closely monitored.

PROBLEMS OVER TAKING MEDICATION

Some patients are not helped despite very large doses of medication, and despite trying a whole range of different ones. Others need to continue to take it for long periods of time without any obvious benefit, but in order to prevent a recurrence of problems. In the early stages it is usually not possible to tell how a given person will respond to drug treatment, or how long they will need to take it. The doctor will keep a close eye on medication, and may vary it from time to time to allow for this.

Occasionally, you or your relative may feel the doctor is issuing repeat prescriptions without assessing the need for them properly. This impression may be a true one, but sometimes arises because of a lack of communication. In either case, it is reasonable for you to seek an opportunity to express your concern to the doctor in order to clarify the situation.

It is difficult for all concerned if someone refuses to take prescribed medication. It may not be possible to convince a reluctant person that medication is helpful until it has had some effect and they are sufficiently improved to notice. People with bipolar disorder may refuse to take lithium because they actually miss feeling 'high'. Hopefully, with support from relatives, a sympathetic doctor will be able to work out the best and most acceptable drug dosage. This can often be gradually reduced as the patient improves.

It may happen that you suspect that your relative is not telling the truth about taking their tablets. In this difficult situation, it is probably not a good idea to confront them immediately. One reasonable course of action is to accompany them to their next appointment with a member of the clinical team. Ask to see the team member separately, and explain the problem. Alternatively, you could do this over the phone. Suggest you might supervise your relative's drug treatment to some extent. To do this, you obviously need to be very clear about the correct dosage, when the medication is to be taken, and the likelihood of any side effects. You can then tell your relative the clinical staff want you to help with medication. Remind your relative when the tablets are due, and watch as he or she takes them. Having established, to some extent, your right to take an interest in this way, it may then also be possible to raise the question of the tablet you find down the toilet, or of the bottle fuller than it ought to be. How you handle this obviously depends on your relationship and whether the necessary frankness can be tolerated. It will not be useful if all you manage to change is the method of disposal.

PSYCHOLOGICAL AND SOCIAL TREATMENTS

While people are in hospital, and frequently after they return home, they will usually be offered some form of psychological treatment or social intervention. This can involve organising various aspects of the environment in the most beneficial way, or individual treatment, or both. There are several ways of doing this, depending on the precise facilities available locally, and also to some extent on the views of local clinical staff about its usefulness for a particular individual.

As we described above, severe mental health problems not only have obvious effects such as suicidal ideas, hallucinations and delusions, but less obvious and more persistent ones. These can cause equally difficult problems. Unlike a straightforward physical condition such as a broken leg or pneumonia, which people can observe and understand relatively easily, those suffering from severe mental illness usually look perfectly normal. This can make it hard for others, and indeed even the individual, to appreciate the unseen difficulties that may continue. These less obvious problems revolve around the negative symptoms, described on page 38, such as slowness, poor concentration, tiredness, underactivity, loss of confidence in one's abilities, loss of interest in previous hobbies or friends, and an inability to show one's feelings. This may mean that your relative does not want, and is not immediately able, to return to a demanding career or a full family life and responsibilities. Social treatments are designed to help in overcoming these difficulties by providing a setting where people can be gradually encouraged to return to a previous level of outside interest and function. It is important for all those concerned with the person's wellbeing to appreciate the special and unforeseen problems that this transition can entail.

Occupational therapy (see also page 81)
Most NHS hospitals have occupational therapy (OT) departments, and some community mental health teams will include an occupational therapist, although these days there are severe shortages, and it is less common to meet one outside of the ward. OT offers a range of activities that will help people to regain lost interests, skills and concentration, while allowing them to feel that their time is creatively and usefully employed during the day. These activities may be organised on a ward, in a day hospital, in a hostel, or at home. Service users can find it helpful to have some structure to their day, and to have somewhere to go to. The activities offered may at first sight look much too simple and undemanding both to you and to your relative. This is because it may be hard, indeed even quite a shock, to realise how poor their concentration and interest

has become. The activities are, in fact, carefully graded to the individual's current capacity. The aim is to help people to regain skills and confidence steadily and gradually, and to minimise the risk of failure which can be very discouraging. People will usually be provided with more complex and demanding tasks when they become capable of them. Sometimes the OT department will encourage totally new interests, such as pottery, art, crafts or cookery, which clients can continue to develop. Your encouragement can be very valuable here.

Many of the activities centre on useful occupational or domestic skills that can be employed to get someone back into the routine of looking after themselves. These are particularly important when someone has been unwell for a appreciable period. Art and crafts are used to stimulate the person and permit a sense of creative achievement. Music, drama and dance may be used to enable them to express themselves. Cooking is always useful.

Tony was an intelligent man who had been admitted to hospital because of a severe depression. Because of this, he had little energy and could hardly be bothered to do anything. His psychiatrist and occupational therapist together worked out a daily programme with him. This was designed in such a way that he was encouraged to use what concentration he could muster, but very little pressure was put on him. Three of his sessions were in the pottery department, where it was suggested that he tried his hand at making relatively small simple objects. He also helped with moving finished pottery around and doing other small tasks. Clearly the occupational therapist did not actually need his help in this way, but she kept him close by her for much of the time, encouraging him, talking to him and organising him. When he returned to the ward, he had the small satisfaction of having done something constructive, however trifling. This was the first stage in a plan to help Tony regain confidence and interest, and as he got better he was gradually led into doing more.

Getting back to work
In the past, mental health staff, and indeed service users themselves, often preferred a more industrial setting to re-establish confidence and concentration and to assist the return to work. Sheltered

workshops were useful for people who had continuing problems. As with occupational therapy, it could be helpful just for the person to have a set timetable, and to have things to do and think about. Working alongside someone else could be beneficial, actually working with someone more so. Once more, the range of jobs, packing or light industrial work, might have looked far too simple, but was graded to the individual's capacity at the time. Occupational and sheltered work used to be the start of a return to full time employment.

However, although these facilities do still exist in some places, access to them became reduced during the 1990s. It was felt that such industrial work was old-fashioned, and in any case most people in work these days are employed in other sectors. The emphasis has now shifted to enabling people to regain lost skills, or to learn new skills if their previous work record was poor. Considerable emphasis is now put on helping people access educational and leisure courses, not just work related activities. These are often very helpful, can be phased in, starting with one or two hours a week, and can develop gradually into full time. Courses and part time sheltered work provide an environment where people can get used to a routine and have interesting things to do each day, and lead to improvements in self esteem and confidence. They also provide an opportunity to meet others and reduce social isolation. This may lead to a return to work but can be rewarding in itself.

Patrick had suffered from a series of depressive illnesses and was also rather obsessive in his habits. This made him slow, if very sure, in any task he might undertake. 'Slow but sure' are not qualities suited to the needs of most jobs these days, and he never managed to stay in work for very long. Recent years had seen him unemployed for most of the time. This did not help his tendency to depression or his relationship with his ageing parents with whom he lived. Eventually, it was decided to offer him a place in a sheltered workshop. He tried out a number of tasks: the one that most suited him had become available only recently in the workshop, and consisted of entering statistical information onto computer discs. Patrick's slowness did not matter too much here and his accuracy was appreciated. It did not seem likely that he would ever work in open employment of this type, but he had his place in the workshop and was much more cheerful. His parents appreciated the fact that he was no longer moping around the house in the daytime, and family life was much easier.

In Patrick's case, sheltered work had an important part in preventing an enduring and serious mental problem from getting worse, and helped him to continue to live in the community. Nowadays most sheltered workshops are run by charities, and may be linked into day care. Local provision of these is therefore variable and there may not be easy access to one in your area.

Group meetings
Day care centres, or drop in facilities organise regular meetings between staff and service users where problems and experiences, both past and present, may be discussed. While some service users say that they find such meetings uncomfortable or boring, others find it very valuable to be able to talk to or listen to others who understand their problems and have shared some of the same experiences. In some settings, meetings are regarded as a central part of treatment. Attention will be focussed on events that happened in childhood, in the belief that these are of crucial importance to the development of current problems. It is then more likely to be referred to as group therapy. Groups in other settings may involve a more direct focus on everyday problems and how to solve them.

Psychological treatment: Individual sessions
Some people will be offered time on their own with clinical staff to discuss their difficulties. As health professionals in the community now tend to work in teams, the staff member involved may be from any one of the variety of professions described on page . The sort of individual therapy offered can be extremely varied, from counselling about recent problems or specific programmes to help modify particular difficulties directly, to detailed sessions in which the relationship between earlier experiences and current problems is explored.

Sometimes only a few sessions are offered, in other cases, weekly sessions over several months or a year or two. The sort of help to be provided should be negotiated and agreed between the service user and the staff at the time. This treatment can be a great help to some people, by getting them to understand what has happened to them, how to prevent it happening again and how to cope in the future, should problems recur.

The regular opportunity to talk privately with a member of the clinical staff is often referred to as 'individual psychotherapy', or just psychotherapy for short. Another name is 'talking therapy'. This takes a whole range of forms and the procedure used by particular practitioners may follow quite closely from their adherence to a chosen theory of human psychology.

Psychoanalysis is a special type of psychotherapy, carried out along lines dictated by the beliefs of psychoanalytic theory. Psychoanalysts have always tended to form splinter groups, each with a different if related theory – so you get Freudian analysts, Jungian analysts, Kleinian analysts, and so forth. All however share the opinion that earlier experiences determine later mental problems in a rather precise way.

Psychoanalysis started, as is well known, in central Europe, but has been most influential in the United States, although its popularity there has waned considerably over the last 30 years. There have been some well known British practitioners, but by and large most British psychiatrists are rather suspicious of elaborate theories that are supported by doubtful evidence. They prefer to keep things relatively simple, and will only take as a fact what has been clearly established. They have been readier to accept biological ideas than psychological ones, probably as a consequence of their medical training. In psychological matters, they are more influenced by the rather different theories of their clinical psychologist colleagues.

Members of the public often don't realise this, and are rather surprised to find that psychiatrists are more concerned with current practical difficulties than with probing the deep recesses of the mind. There is no doubt about the past influence of psychoanalytic ideas, and psychiatrists readily recognise that early experiences are likely to be important in shaping the way people behave in adult life. However, they tend to think that not a lot can be done to change what has already happened. Psychoanalysts, in contrast, think that very early experience can affect later life by influencing it in ways that individual does not know about, and that bringing these influence into consciousness can help to repair them.

However, most psychotherapy carried out in the National Health Service is 'supportive psychotherapy', concentrating on everyday problems, although with some attempt to give the patient insight

into their behaviour. Clinical psychologists may offer psychotherapy of this type, but also provide special types, most commonly
'cognitive behavioural therapy'.

Cognitive Behaviour Therapy (CBT)
The adjective 'cognitive' refers to thought, and cognitive therapy is
based on the idea that people's emotional states depend upon their
thinking. Depressed people are locked into a gloomy misinterpretation
of events and the light they cast on themselves. These thoughts have
become automatic and therefore difficult to shift eg. 'I am useless',
'My life is not worth living'. The therapist starts by discussing these
thinking styles, and helps the person become more aware: how you
think can influence directly how you feel. Making these processes
more apparent gives someone the chance of 'rethinking' or distancing
themselves from this thinking, and perhaps replacing it with more
positive ideas. 'My thoughts are just thoughts. It's not true that I am
useless'. This newer treatment is effective in treating depression and
also keeps it at bay once people have recovered, as they can themselves
begin to identify these patterns and deal with them earlier.

In the last 15 years, cognitive behaviour therapy (CBT) has
developed from a successful approach to depression and anxiety to
one that has been applied equally successfully to psychosis. You
may have heard of 'CBT for psychosis'. It had been thought for
many years that, because delusional ideas are often held with great
conviction, it was impossible to change them by discussion. Thus
'talking therapies' were not offered to people with psychosis, and
treatment concentrated on medication and the various social
interventions we have discussed above. However evidence is now
accumulating that by helping people to review the evidence for their
beliefs, in a sympathetic and non confrontative way, even very fixed
ideas can begin to shift. This treatment is not yet generally
available. However as it was recommended in the NICE Guidelines
for Schizophrenia and the evidence for its effectiveness is now
good, many clinicians are currently learning about it and are
interested in trying to offer it. Sessions are usually offered at least
fortnightly over six months.

Counselling
This is another increasingly available talking therapy. The term is
not well defined, and can cover a range of approaches from

supportive listening to sophisticated help with dealing with difficulties. Counselling is usually short-term, and rarely offered to those with severe mental health problems, but is increasingly available at GP's surgeries, health centres and privately. Either you or your relative may find it useful to have an outside person to offer you support. Your relative should be able to obtain problem solving and emotional support, as well as practical help from their care coordinator.

Family intervention
This form of psycho-social treatment, or psychological treatment as it is now called was developed in the 1970's. Whole families are asked to meet together with one, or sometimes two, professional staff to discuss areas of difficulty. This form of treatment is appropriate if the service users are in close contact with their family, as their relatives are then likely to continue to be involved in their care. Family meetings will be offered by staff as individual circumstances dictate: they may be limited to one or two occasions, or continue over some months or years. Some families find it extremely useful to look at how they get on together, to understand why difficulties have occurred in the past and to consider how they might help each other cope with problems. A particular kind of psychosocial family work has been developed, both in the UK and the USA, which deals with the problems routinely found when carers have to deal with psychosis in the family. This has been shown to be very effective in helping clients recover and to stay well, and in helping carers to cope better with longstanding problems. Again it has been recommended by the NICE Guidelines particularly when carer and service user are in close contact and when the service user continues to have new episodes and continuing symptoms. This might be available from your local mental health team, at least for a few families. As a carer you are entitled to a yearly carer assessment and as part of this you can ask for some family sessions if this would be helpful.

Carer groups
Most relatives' groups are self help groups organised by interested relatives to enable them to share problems and support each other. RETHINK is the best known of these organisations in the UK and is worth describing in some detail – you may find what it offers is

useful to you. Details of its excellent website are given in the appendix at the end of the book. It used to be called the National Schizophrenia Fellowship.

RETHINK offers a variety of services to carers and service users. Obviously, some of these are more or less restricted to those who become members of the organisation. Participation in local RETHINK groups provides information about local services but also, more importantly perhaps, personal support and the exchange of information about problems of caring. Membership also gives access to various projects the local groups may have set up. One of their most successful recent initiatives has been to offer carer led groups for several meetings, Carer Educational and Support for Psychosis (CESP). These are a mixture of educational and emotional support, and have been found very helpful by carers. Carers' groups run fortnightly for about 10 sessions. There will probably be one running in your local area. It can be enormously helpful to share difficulties and solutions with other carers who know what the problems can be.

Other support includes social events, respite holidays, housing, sheltered employment, social clubs, day centres and benefits. The group can provide 'muscle' to back up individual member's dissatisfactions or complaints. There is also the facility of telephoning knowledgeable RETHINK members in local areas, and a 24-hour help line is available.

In addition, RETHINK headquarters also offers an advisory service, which is available to all. There is also a library of video and audio-tapes covering much of current expert opinion about schizophrenia. There are lists of publications helpful to relatives, some of which are produced by RETHINK itself.

Advice is available about complaints procedures. Indeed Rethink will take up specific problems with the statutory service if your own attempts have been unsuccessful. This service is limited by the availability of personnel, and so may give priority to actual members. The sorts of problem that RETHINK often has to deal with are the threatened or actual discharge home of a still unwell person to a relative who cannot cope, the refusal of hospital admission to a very disturbed person at home, lack of information about medication and its likely side effects, an inadequate service from the family doctor, and general dissatisfaction with psychiatrist services or the mental health team. RETHINK also represents relatives' and carers' views to policy makers and service providers (Commissioners, Health Authorities, Local Authorities, Government, professional bodies). They campaign and lobby on issues brought to their attention by relatives.

The Manic Depression Fellowship is an organization for those who suffer from manic depressive illness and their relatives (see appendix). For a small annual fee, it offers to members a quarterly newsletter, occasional fact sheets, meetings and perhaps most especially, assistance in setting up local self-help groups. Compared with RETHINK, a larger proportion of members are service users.

Mind's local associations sometimes can and do act as support groups for troubled relatives, as well as providing a range of helpful support to service users.

ALTERNATIVE MEDICINE AND PSYCHIATRY

You may come across other treatments for which claims are made, such as special diets or regimes. Distressed people and their relatives may be dissatisfied with their response to routine therapy, particularly if it doesn't seem to improve things much. They are sometimes therefore willing to place their faith in something that appears to offer an alternative. Unfortunately, such treatments are sometimes proposed by uncritical enthusiasts, and sometimes by those with a strong financial interest in promoting them.

Practitioners in this area are now organising themselves into societies that will establish standards of practice and methods of investigating the effectiveness of any new treatment. Nevertheless, we have considerable reservations, and feel that carers should be cautious about unconventional treatments with limited evidence of effectiveness.

6 Looking After Yourself

COPING WITH YOURSELF

This may not seem an obvious aspect for you to be concerned about, and it is easily overlooked. The focus may be so much on your relative, severely mentally unwell and vulnerable, that your own feelings or problems can be forgotten or not recognised. This is a great pity, and indeed one of the reasons for this book.

Living and coping with an individual who has had a severe mental illness can be rewarding, with no particular problems. Often, however, this is not the case, particularly at first, and your own reactions may be crucial to your ability to deal with problems effectively and to prevent crises from developing. Individuals with some severe mental illnesses, particularly schizophrenia, can be especially sensitive to the family atmosphere. If you are able to cope effectively with the difficulties that arise, tension will be reduced, arguments avoided, and problems lessened.

The first important thing to be learned is that it is in everyone's interest for you to try to deal with difficulties calmly and with tolerance, even if you aren't feeling particularly calm. This helps people to recover more quickly and indeed keeps them well.

For example, a sister who was living with her twin who had become ill, described how initially she had been very impatient and irritated by her behaviour, particularly her inability to do various things, or help around the house. As time passed however she realised that this attitude was making things worse. She said 'I realised it was no good, so I learned to be more patient'. This was without anyone's advice or help, she just learned with the passage of time that some things were helpful, and other things made life harder. This more patient and tolerant attitude, expecting a little less and not becoming so angry, made the atmosphere much calmer between them, and helped her sister to recover.

The second important principle that may help you cope is that you need to have your own interests and to lead your own life if you wish to. It is quite possible to be extremely caring and supportive whilst maintaining your own outside interests, going to work and going on holiday. People very often feel they should give all of this up: it is natural to feel that you should not leave your relative alone at home just to go out and enjoy yourself. However, this seems to be a mistake. Carers who are able to lead their own lives to some extent and who do not become totally immersed in looking after their relative, do feel better themselves. However, very crucially, they are also able to allow the person a degree of independence. In our experience, relatives who have lived with mentally ill people for many years very rarely have a holiday. However, if they start going out sometimes, perhaps going to work even, if only part-time, or doing other things by themselves and for themselves, this can restore the balance and reduce the tendency to do too much for the other person, rather than just enough.

One couple were very worried that, if they left their son alone in the house for any length of time, he would set fire to the kitchen while making himself a cup of tea. In fact this had nearly happened on several occasions in the past, so it was not an unrealistic fear. However, after safeguarding the kitchen as much as possible beforehand, they tried a few hours away from home. No disaster happened, and it was possible to build on this in order to restore some of this couple's own life and enjoyment together.

Related to the necessity of doing things for your own satisfaction (and in the process allowing your relative some independence), is the danger of being too protective. People with severe mental illness are usually adults, even if they have not all managed to achieve much independent adult life. It can be too easy to go back to treating them as children: unable to be left alone, to look after themselves or to make their own decisions. It is quite true that at various stages of their severe mental health problems, people may lose the ability to look after themselves properly, or lose contact with reality and not care about such things. However this state is not usually permanent, and it is all too easy for you to get into the habit of doing and organising all the things that need to be done.

In one family, Carl was able to cook a meal and do some cleaning and shopping, but it was easier and more efficient for his 70 year old mother to do it all for both of them. It took some time and effort to establish that Carl should do more than he did round the house, and to decide that he should be responsible for at least one meal a week. Once this was achieved it was possible to build on it, so that Carl felt that he had achieved something and was of some use around the house, and his mother could begin to share some of the responsibilities she had always taken on alone.

The third important principle in coping with mental illness in the family is to avoid being too intrusive. It is of course not a good idea to leave your ill relative totally alone and isolated, particularly as these illnesses have in any case a tendency to make the sufferer withdraw from other people. However, it is also useful to know when to leave someone alone. One mother said 'I follow him around the house, I'm so worried what he'll do next'. While it is understandable and natural to worry, and while it may be necessary at times of acute illness to be very observant, for instance when there is a risk of suicide, this level of worry, anger or upset can continue even when things are a little better. At this stage it can be very wearing and quite destructive for you, if you have no relief. It may also prevent you developing more tolerant and realistic attitudes. It is often desirable for the person to be able to go and lie down in their own room for a while, as they may frequently be over-sensitive to the presence of other people and feel they simply have to be left alone sometimes. One mother said, 'I know he gets upset at times and he goes to his bedroom. I don't go in for a while, just leave him, then later on, I'll offer him a cup of tea, take it in to him if he won't come down, and ask if things are any better'. One man's inactivity made his wife very angry, as she had to take on all the household chores, child care and a part-time job. She said 'Sometimes I just go for a walk round the park to get away from him for a while. It means I can calm down and feel better when I go back in'.

Those who cope successfully with the problems have usually come to recognise both what is helpful and what is not. It often happens that their expectations of their relative's future performance or life style have to change. It can be tragic to watch a much loved son or daughter fall short of early hopes, or to see a partner not able to match up to the initial promise of a relationship. Many parents and spouses talk of a time similar to that following bereavement and equally painful, when these adjustments take place in their hopes and expectations. It does of course help to be tactful about sharing these feelings with the person involved.

Particularly if you are a partner, you are likely at one time or another to feel that you want to end the relationship. This may be realistic and probably happens to every couple at some stage. In some cases it is the best outcome, and individuals and their families manage better with less frequent and less intense contact, particularly if this has been very upsetting in the past. Professionals often suggest that grown-up children do not return home to live full time with their parents but go to a hostel, or sheltered housing, or their own flat. It may be a better and much more realistic long term solution to keep in a degree of contact of your own choosing with a relative living elsewhere, than to be forced to continue to live together when problems have become insurmountable. Such decisions are best made after discussion between you, your relative and their key-worker.

For some people, the only compensation for caring for their relative comes from a sense of duty done. While this deserves respect, it should not blind them to what may be best for the person where, for example, home circumstances are so fraught that separation would be the best answer. Those who feel there are few rewards for caring should try to make sure that other aspects of their lives compensate. One carer wisely advises, 'in order to cope with sometimes unbearable strain, you must keep well, eat well, get as much sleep and exercise as you can. Try to keep up with your work and hobbies, and try to find support in what you can – religion, friendship, a sense of mission. Do not hide your difficulties from relatives and friends: if you do, they will think you do not need their sympathy'.

THE FUTURE

You may be able to retain an optimistic attitude to the future, to view things calmly and deal with problems as they arise. On the other hand you may well feel pessimistic, see no way of changing things and expect grave and insoluble problems to persist. These attitudes do tend to be self fulfilling.

If your relative can accept treatment from clinical staff, if you encourage this and remain calm about crises, and if there are few additional problems such as financial hardship, an initially fraught situation may eventually become acceptable, routine and even quite satisfying. Then you may worry about becoming older: 'What will happen when I am gone?' This is often a realistic fear, as many caring relatives, particularly parents, provide such high levels of support they cannot be replaced. Ideally, part of the care that you provide should aim to enable your relative (as any other adult) to become as independent as possible. Keeping links with other family members and friends may be important for you, but also ensures your relative has others to turn to at times. It is also sensible to make sure your relative does not lose domestic skills or the ability to look after themselves. Help with this is often provided by community occupational therapists who may visit your home and your relative should be encouraged to do this.

It is important to remember that in time most people either recover from their illness or become adapted to its effects. Individual may learn what can upset them and begin to avoid it, or reduce its effects in other ways. With sympathetic care, they may come to accept that medication has a useful role to play in the control of their illness and to comply with a dosage that has the fewest possible side effects. Some people will recover completely. Others will eventually be able to reduce or stop medication. In time, you and your relative can often become adept at recognising the warning signs of an impending relapse and mobilising prompt treatment for it, thus reducing the length and upset of later bouts of illness. Some individuals and their carers are also able to say that such illnesses provide experiences other people can never have, and have added to their lives in unexpectedly fulfilling ways.

HOLIDAYS

These can be a very important source of relief for people living with someone suffering from a mental illness. After all, it can be a full-time job, and any other sort of worker is entitled to periods of leave. Separate holidays are the ideal, at least on occasion, and you shouldn't feel guilty about this – it also gives your relative a break from you!

Some social services departments will organise holidays for mentally ill people, and you may find out about other possibilities from the Psychiatric Rehabilitation Association or the Holiday Care Service (see appendix). Your relative may lack the energy or motivation to do this, so you may have to arrange the holiday for them. It may be possible to get financial help if you and your relative are on a low income.

You may feel it is difficult to go off on holiday on your own. Sometimes, this feeling may be misplaced: your relative might well be able, and indeed happy, to manage on their own for a week or two. Sometimes, it may be realistic for you to feel that they couldn't manage. In such circumstances, you might be able to persuade another relative, either to come and stay, or to have your relative to stay with them while you are on holiday. You may need to make it clear that it is not a permanent arrangement! In some cases, your relative's mental health team may be sympathetic and arrange, say, a fortnight's respite care so you can go on holiday – after all, this is a very efficient use of services, to support someone undertaking much of the responsibility for caring for a mentally ill person. In some areas local charities such as the RETHINK provide this facility.

GETTING FURTHER ADVICE AND INFORMATION

We have mentioned many of these sources of support already.

Information about your local NHS facilities will be available from your family doctor, although even these days some are less well informed than they might be. The mental health team dealing with your relative are perhaps a more reliable source, and the team's linked social worker, or the 'duty' social worker at social services might be the best person to contact. One way of finding out about the available facilities is to ask at the discharge planning meeting.

Other agencies that provide information about local facilities include the local social services departments, the Citizen's Advice Bureau, the Community Health Council, and your local branch of Mind.

Information about employment for the mentally ill can be obtained from the Disablement Resettlement Officer at your local job centre, who will also know about facilities for employment rehabilitation.

RETHINK can be a great source of support as well as of information (see also page 133). Mind (the National Association for Mental Health) is very good at meeting requests for information, and have a range of booklets about particular topics. The Mental Health Foundation, who commissioned the first edition of this book, also have booklets and publications concerning related subjects. Several books give information about financial benefits. These include the 'Disability Rights Handbook' of the Disability

Alliance Educational and Research Association, and the 'National Welfare Benefits Handbook' and 'Rights Guide to non Means Tested Social Security Benefits' published by the Child Poverty Action Group.

The names and addresses of over 10,000 'self help' and community organisations in the United Kingdom both national and local, are published by the Mental Health Foundation in their 'Someone to Talk to Directory', available through your local library. It might be worth your while to look at this.

Another useful source of information is the Institute of Psychiatry, KCL, which publishes the latest research, together with stories from carers at www.mentalhealthcare.org.uk. The British Psychological Society publishes the latest psychological research on the causes, experiences and treatment of psychosis: www.understandingpsychosis.com.

7 Legal Matters

The most important part of this chapter deals with the rules which have to be followed in arranging compulsory admission and compulsory treatment, and the safeguards that exist. Since we wrote the first edition of this book, it has become much harder to get admitted to hospital because of the reduction in acute beds. As a result, people are often admitted in the later stages of a crisis and so a higher proportion of admissions are on a compulsory basis, around 20% in the services we work in. Sadly therefore, an appreciable number of our readers will require information about compulsory admission, and we have given it in some detail. Rather than summarise all the mental health legislation, we have concentrated on those parts most likely to be relevant to people who suffer from schizophrenia and manic depressive illness.

THE RIGHTS OF PATIENTS AND RELATIVES

Most admissions to hospital happen because clients agree with members of the mental health team that this is the best way to deal with their difficulties. This is known as informal or voluntary admission. When admission is thought to be necessary, people are always given the opportunity to agree to it. Sometimes, however, they may need to be admitted to, or detained in, hospital against their will. In Britain, we have always been careful to defend the rights of individuals, and compulsory admission is a legal process with legal safeguards. The law in England and Wales is based on the 1983 Mental Health Act. Under this Act, the nearest relative of a compulsorily detained patient has both rights and duties, and may be involved in the admission procedure. Acts along similar lines apply in Scotland and Northern Ireland.

THE RIGHTS OF VOLUNTARY PATIENTS

Voluntary admission to hospital is by mutual agreement of the client and of the clinical team. Under these circumstances, clients have the right to refuse treatment and to discharge themselves. However, if your relative refuses to work with the clinical team to establish a mutually agreed plan of treatment, this will make it very difficult for the team to help them. Situations like this may even cause difficulties for the treatment of other patients in the ward. It is much better to try to discuss disagreements with staff in order to find an acceptable solution. In extreme cases, the team may decide to discharge clients if they are not cooperating with plans for treatment, on the grounds that care in hospital has ceased to be of benefit. Even in such cases they should offer some kind of alternative provision, particularly where the patient is clearly suffering from the consequences of a severe mental illness like schizophrenia or manic depressive illness.

If clients do decide that they want to discharge themselves against medical advice, they may be asked to sign a statement to that effect. This might be used in the light of subsequent developments to protect the clinical team from allegations of negligence.

In some cases, people agree to be admitted on a voluntary basis even though they may be seriously disturbed and a potential danger to themselves or others. If they then change their mind and want to discharge themselves, the medical team may well decide that they must remain in the hospital on a compulsory basis. Staff feel required to do this when they think their duty of care outweighs the obligation to treat people by mutual agreement where at all possible. Patients may feel this is a betrayal of the original agreement, although it should only happen when staff are very worried about the situation. In other cases, someone may deteriorate in hospital despite the attentions of staff, and this may also lead the team to consider compulsory detention, particularly if they are refusing a needed treatment. This state of affairs does give considerable powers to psychiatrists and social workers, which you and your relative may feel uneasy about. In most cases the powers are used for the genuine benefit of the client, and there are safeguards, which we describe below.

THE PATIENT'S NEAREST RELATIVE

The nearest relative is the one the client usually lived with or who was most involved in caring for them before going into hospital. Where there is more than one such person or the client lives alone, the legal nearest relative is the one closest to the top of the list in Table 9.

TABLE 9
Nearest relatives

husband/wife
son/daughter
father/mother
brother/sister
grandparent
grandchild
uncle/aunt
nephew/niece

A cohabitee may qualify as nearest relative if they have lived with the client for at least six months as husband or wife. They do not however take over the rights of the actual husband or wife unless there has been a legal separation or divorce. A person other than a relative who has lived with the client for at least five years counts as a relative but in the last position on the list.

WHO CAN BE ADMITTED OR DETAINED AGAINST THEIR WILL?

Compulsory procedures can only be used to admit or detain clients suffering from certain types of disorder. The rules governing this are laid down in the 1983 Act. The person must be suffering from a mental disorder sufficiently severe to make admission appropriate and must have refused voluntary admission. The admission must be in the interests of the client's own health or safety, or for the protection of others. 'Mental disorder' covers three conditions; mental illness, psychopathic disorder, and mental impairment (learning disability); but excludes sexual deviation and dependence on alcohol or drugs. Slightly different powers apply to each of these three conditions. Those suffering from 'mental illness' are subject to the widest powers. The British Acts do not define what is meant by this term, although the Northern Irish one does, but it would clearly cover both schizophrenia and manic depressive illness. Compulsory admission is most commonly used for suicidal clients, for those who act on beliefs of persecution, and for those who are incapable of looking after themselves physically or who may cause themselves untold social damage, running up huge debts and the like.

ADMISSION AND DETENTION UNDER THE MENTAL HEALTH ACT

There are different sections of the Act describing the proper procedures for use in particular circumstances. The duration of detention varies according to the procedure used, and the recommendation for detention can be renewed when it runs out. There are particular rules for clients admitted following criminal proceedings that are not discussed here.

Under Section 136 of the Act, people suspected of being a danger to themselves or others and found in a public place can be taken to a *place of safety* by a police officer. These powers are used with increasing frequency, but are usually monitored by a committee with representatives from the police and the local mental health Trust. Usually, a place of safety means a hospital, making it relatively easy for the client to be assessed by a doctor and an approved social worker. This must be done within 72 hours. A place of safety can mean a residential home or a police station, but these are less suitable and less commonly used.

Under Section 135, an approved social worker can apply to a Magistrate to issue a warrant for premises to be searched for someone suspected to be mentally disordered. There must be grounds for believing that they are being mistreated or neglected, or are alone and unable to care for themselves. The warrant is carried out by a police officer, accompanied by a social worker and a doctor.

However, these circumstances are relatively unusual. A commoner situation arises when, because of a disturbance indoors, at home or elsewhere, someone calls the family doctor, who thinks the sufferer should be admitted but cannot persuade him or her to enter hospital voluntarily. The procedure then requires an *application*, which can be signed either by a specially approved social worker or by the nearest relative. There also has to be one or more *medical recommendations*. If there is only one such recommendation, this permits an *emergency admission*, under Section 4 of the Act. In this case the medical recommendation should preferably be from a doctor who knows the person, most usually their GP. The client can only be held for 72 hours, unless another doctor is obtained within this period to make an additional recommendation, thus converting it to a Section 2 admission (see below). A social worker signing the application form without the knowledge of the nearest relative must, with all urgency, tell the relative what has happened. Both the doctor and the social worker must have seen the client within 24 hours of signing their part of the Section. Thus the decision to Section is based primarily on how the person is on that day, and previous problems, however worrying, do not always get taken into consideration, if they are not current.

Admission for assessment requires the recommendation of two doctors, and one of them must be recognised as having special psychiatric expertise. This type of admission is permitted by Section 2 of the Act, and the compulsory power lasts for 28 days. The guidelines to the act make it clear that Section 2 permits compulsory treatment by physical methods like drugs or ECT.

Clients who have been admitted compulsorily can be stopped from leaving the hospital by staff, and if they do leave they can be brought back. This provision has been changed in the Mental Health (Patients in the Community) Act of 1995. Patients on Sections, and some other Sections imposed by courts, can be brought back at anytime up to 6 months or, if later, the end of the existing authority for detention. If they are not brought back within this period, however, this power is lost.

Although people can be treated under Section 2, Section 3 of the Act refers specifically to *admission for treatment*. The power to detain lasts for up to six months, but can then be renewed for a further six months. After that it can be renewed annually. Under Section 3, if the nearest relative objects, the social worker cannot make the application. However, if the social worker thinks the relative is being unreasonable, they may apply to a County Court for the nearest relative's function to be transferred to someone else, who need not be another relative. The guidelines to the 1983 Act emphasise that where a patient is known to the mental health team, Section 3 is more appropriate than Section 2.

There may be circumstances in which you may feel your relative needs compulsory admission. One way of doing this is by calling the family doctor, and yourself signing the application. Another way is to ask the local social services department to arrange for an approved social worker to consider the case. If satisfied that compulsory admission cannot be avoided, the social worker will then make an application under the Act. If the social worker does not think compulsory admission is justified, they must inform you in writing. They are also obliged to consider all other alternatives to compulsory admission.

There are also powers under Section 5 of the Act that can be used by designated doctors and nurses to prevent a client from leaving, even when they originally agreed to go into hospital voluntarily. Once more, it must be thought that the client is a danger to themselves or others. This power to detain is important, because otherwise the client would have to be allowed to leave, and might experience considerable suffering or damage before the procedures of Section 4 could be arranged.

Details of the sections of the 1983 Mental Health Act that govern compulsory admission procedures are summarised in Table 10.

TABLE 10

1983 Mental Health Act Part II: Compulsory admission

Section	Purpose	Applicant	Medical recommendation	Duration	Outcome
4	Emergency assessment (mental disorder)	Nearest relative or approved social worker (who must have seen the patient within the previous 24 hours)	Any doctor	72 hours	Discharge of order: by lapse; by consultant; by managers; by nearest relative. Conversion to Section 2 by second medical recommendation.
2	Assessment (mental disorder)	Nearest relative or approved social worker who must attempt to inform the nearest relative	Two doctors, one approved under the Mental Health Act as having special expertise in psychiatry	28 days	Discharge of order: by lapse; by consultant; by managers; by nearest relative. Conversion to Section 3.
3	Treatment (i) Mental illness or severe mental impairment (ii) Psychopathic disorder or mental impairment if treatable	Nearest relative or approved social worker, provided that he has attempted to consult the nearest relative who must consent.	Two doctors, as above, giving reasons for detention, form of disorder and consideration of other methods of g dealing with the patient	6 months renewable for a further 6 months then at yearly intervals	Discharge of order: by lapse; by consultant; by managers; by nearest relative. By MHRT.

SAFEGUARDS FOLLOWING A COMPULSORY ADMISSION

It is possible for the compulsory powers to be revoked before they run out, and indeed this is the commonest outcome for Section 3. This is usually done by the doctor in charge of the client, the *Responsible Medical Officer* or RMO. For instance, the doctor may revoke an emergency section (Section 4), feeling that although it was a reasonable course of action at the time, it now looks to have been inappropriately applied. In other cases, the client has asked for the compulsory order to be suspended. They may be considerably better and in any case likely to be reasonably cooperative with treatment, either as an informal inpatient or as an outpatient. The original requirements for the Section now no longer apply. In such cases, the doctor will often be happy to agree, feeling that treatment by mutual consent is more pleasant and more likely to be effective.

The *Hospital Managers* can also revoke compulsory powers. These people should not be confused with the management of the hospital. They are lay people, and the panel may include non-executive directors of the hospital trust and coopted or associate members. Clients can appeal directly to the hospital managers to discharge them, and do not need any one's permission to do this. A Managers' Hearing will then be arranged, and the panel may confirm the client's discharge. Clients may also ask for a solicitor to represent them.

If a client is discharged from compulsory detention, the nearest relative must be informed, unless either they or the client have requested otherwise.

Clients also have the right to appear before a *Mental Health Review Tribunal (MHRT)*, which may order their release. The Hospital Managers have a duty to inform compulsorily detained clients about their rights and, in particular, about their right of appeal to these Tribunals. Provided the client agrees, the Managers must also inform the nearest relative of these rights, and in certain cases the relative can also apply to the Tribunal for the client to be reviewed. The application must be in writing. Clients can ask to be represented at the Tribunal by a friend or relative, or by a legal representative. MIND (the National Association for Mental Health – see address list) offers help with

representation. Legal aid is available to all who appeal to the
MHRT, and the representation organised by MIND is also free.

These tribunals are independent bodies that ensure that people
admitted to hospital are not being kept there unnecessarily. Each
National Health Executive in England has one, and there is one
for the whole of Wales. The hearings are conducted by a
president, who is a lawyer, with one medical and one lay
colleague to help. The main duty of tribunals is to decide whether
a person can be released from hospital. They can also order them
to be discharged at some future date. They can compel witnesses
to attend, and take evidence under oath. Hearings are usually in
private, although the client or relative can request a public
hearing.

Clients are only allowed to apply to tribunals at certain
intervals. As you might suspect, there is no right of appeal to the
tribunal where detention is compelled under those sections of the
Act, such as Section 4, that only hold for 72 hours. Details are
given in Tables 11 and 12.

TABLE 11

Periods of eligibility for Mental Health Review Tribunals

Mental Health Act 1983	First 14 days	First 6 months	Second 6 months	Annually
Sections 4, 5, 136 (72 hours)	–	–	–	–
Section 2 (28 days)	✓	–	–	–
Section 3 (treatment order)	–	✓	✓	✓
Section 37 (hospital order)	–	–	✓	✓
Sections 37 and 41 (hospital order with restriction order)	–	–	✓	✓

The right of patients to appeal both to the hospital managers
and to a Mental Health Review Tribunal has sometimes led to a
duplication of procedures, and there are currently plans to
remove the duty of hospital managers to hear appeals.

TABLE 12
Automatic Mental Health Review Tribunals

Mental Health Act 1983	First 6 months	Second 6 months	Every 3 years
Sections 3 (treatment order	–	✓	✓
Section 37 (hospital order)	–	–	✓
Sections 37 and 41 (hospital order with restriction order)	–	–	✓

If you are the nearest relative, you can discharge someone held under the powers of the Mental Health Act. It requires 72 hours notice in writing to the Hospital Managers, so the power obviously doesn't apply to those sections of the Act that only empower detention for 72 hours. The medical officer in charge of treatment can countermand your powers of discharge, but this in turn must be done in writing and you can then refer your relative to a Mental Health Review Tribunal, provided they are not detained under Section 2.

Mind's legal department will always advise you, and the organisation's booklet A Mental Health Review Tribunal May Help You explains how to apply. You should be able to get this from your hospital social worker, the local Community Health Council, the Citizens' Advice Bureau or through Mind itself.

COMPULSORY TREATMENT

In some emergency situations, any client can be given medication under common law without their consent, although the treatment given must be appropriate to the scale of the emergency. Indeed this is actually spelt out by the Mental Health Act for compulsorily detained clients. In other situations, voluntary clients can only be treated if they agree to it: they have the right to refuse under common law. Legal consent to treatment does not just mean agreeing to it. The doctor must explain the nature, purpose and effect of the treatment and the client must be of sound enough mind to understand it. However, there is no formal procedure for obtaining a voluntary client's consent to drug treatment – if they accept the doctor's prescription, it is assumed that this indicates consent. ECT is regarded as the equivalent of a minor operation, and so clients are required to sign a consent form. Where voluntary clients are so mentally disturbed that they cannot understand the nature of the treatment offered, the doctor is really obliged to convert their admission into a compulsory one.

Clients who are compulsorily detained are often able to consent to treatment in the normal way. They can also be treated against their will in certain circumstances. However, ECT and long lasting courses of medicine can only be given with the client's consent or on the strength of an independent second medical opinion, that is, the opinion of a doctor who does not work in the same hospital as the consultant responsible.

Any client can withdraw consent to treatment at any time. The psychiatrist's decision to embark on compulsory treatment of a detained client is then governed by the safeguards of the Mental Health Act. The cases of clients who are being treated compulsorily are monitored by the Mental Health Commission set up under the 1983 Act. This is an independent body made up of legal and medical professionals and lay people and responsible to the Secretary of State. Every three months treatment must be reviewed with the client. If the client can and does give consent to the proposed continuing treatment, the RMO has to sign a form to that effect. Otherwise, the case has to be reviewed by a second opinion doctor provided by the Mental Health Act Commission and only if he or she agrees can treatment proceed.

Members of the commission also visit hospitals at least once or twice a year and ensure the correct working of the 1983 Mental Health Act. At the time a detention order is due for renewal, if treatment has had to be authorised by a second opinion doctor, the doctor in charge of the client's case must report to the Commission on their condition and the progress of treatment. The Commission may itself request such a report at any time, and has the power to withdraw the authority for compulsory treatment, although it cannot discharge patients from detention.

In 1996 there was an addition to the legal powers of psychiatrists brought in under the Mental Health (Patients in the Community) Act. This allows for supervised discharge of certain people detained in hospital under the 1983 Mental Health Act. Most often it relates to people detained under Section 3. The introduction of this legislation has been attended by a lot of public debate. It is a response to concerns about people who do not do well after discharge from hospital because they habitually omit to take medication, to the extent that it is not possible to maintain their care in the community.

However, some people think these powers take too much away from the civil liberty of people with severe mental illness. It is a matter, as with all this legislation, of balancing the right to treatment of people whose mental state prevents cooperation against their right to refuse.

Supervised discharge applies to people who do not need care in hospital any longer, but who would present a substantial risk of serious harm to their own health or safety, or the safety of others, unless their aftercare is supervised. A supervisor, usually the key-worker, is appointed, and has the power to require their client to reside in a specified place and to attend for medical treatment and rehabilitation, and to convey them to a place where they are to attend for occupation, education or treatment. If the arrangements fail, the care team has to review the care plan. At the review the care team should consider whether Compulsory Admission under the 1983 Act is necessary. Clients cannot be given medical treatment in the community against their will. Supervised discharge lasts, initially, six months, but can be extended.

The application for supervised discharge is made by the 'responsible medical officer' while the client is still in hospital under a Section, and should be accompanied by a medical recommendation and a recommendation from an approved social worker.

At the time of writing, we do not yet know if this power will add significantly to the benefit of clients living at home. Psychiatrists may be reluctant to apply it because bad feeling may result and interfere with effective long-term care.

CLIENT'S MAIL

Except for clients in 'special' hospitals like Broadmoor, mail from a client cannot be intercepted unless the person to whom it is addressed has asked for this in writing. The client has to be informed of the interception by the hospital authorities, again in writing. Mail to a client in an ordinary psychiatric hospital cannot be intercepted.

COMPLAINING ABOUT TREATMENT OR THE USE OF COMPULSORY POWERS

You or your relative may complain, either during admission or later, about any aspect of care. In addition to the normal channels open to the citizen (such as writing to Members of Parliament, Ministers of the Crown, the Parliamentary Commissioner, the Health Service Commissioner or the local Community Health Centre) there are three special sources of redress for clients and their relatives. The Hospital Managers should be approached first, and only if you are still not satisfied should you take things further. The Mental Health Review Tribunals have already been mentioned on page . In addition, relatives and clients may apply to the Mental Health Act Commission. The Commission may be contacted by letter, or when members are visiting the hospital. The Commission may deal with a complaint directly, or under certain circumstances by referring it to other procedures set up for the purpose. Clients and relatives can contact the Commission only about procedures under the powers of the Mental Health Act – basically, compulsory admission or treatment. Other complaints should be dealt with through the Hospital Complaints Procedure.

In Scotland and Northern Ireland, the procedures covering compulsory admission and treatment are laid down in separate Acts of Parliament. These are similar in principle to, but differ in detail from, the Mental Health Act that applies in England and Wales. If you live in those areas, you may obtain guidance about the local legislation from local branches of Mind, or from the hospital to which your relative has been admitted.

In Scotland, applications for compulsory admission must be submitted to a Sheriff. There are no Mental Health Review Tribunals, but the Scottish equivalent of the Mental Health Commission, called the Mental Welfare Commission, has responsibility for reviewing and, if appropriate, discharging clients. It also looks after the interests of voluntary clients. The Mental Health Commission for Northern Ireland also has the duty of reviewing the care and treatment of all mentally disordered people. However, it cannot discharge them. This can only be done by the N.I. Mental Health Review Tribunal.

Finally, detained clients can sue for compensation, if the motive for detaining them was improper, or if the doctors were negligent in making their medical recommendations. They can sue anyone involved in the process – the doctors, social workers, nurses, or indeed the nearest relative. However, they need the permission of the High Court to bring a civil action, and of the Director of Public Prosecutions to bring a criminal action.

WILLS AND CONTRACTS

Everyone knows that wills always start off with references to 'being of sound mind'. In fact, the person making the will only has to be of sound enough mind to know what their particular will means. They have to know what property they have, who has a claim on it, and what the relative strengths of their claims are. The will must be legible and unambiguous. Solicitors may seek medical opinion on their client's state of mind.

Contracts require a sound mind in the same way that wills do. Marriage is a contract and in theory would be void if one of the partners was at the time incapable of understanding the nature and responsibilities of marriage. More usually marriages are regarded as voidable, not because a partner was incapable of giving consent, but because they were suffering from a mental disorder of such a nature and extent as to unfit them for marriage. In practice this procedure is rarely used.

OTHER RIGHTS AND DUTIES

For most people admission to hospital is temporary and they can vote as from their home address. For clients staying longer a general hospital or nursing home can be used as an address for the purposes of the electoral roll. However, a mental hospital is not a valid address. Compulsory clients who do not have a place of residence outside the hospital cannot vote.

People seeing a doctor for treatment of a mental illness are excused jury service.

If someone becomes aware of any disability that is likely to affect their ability to drive, they are obliged to inform the Driver and Vehicle Licensing Agency. Mental illness is such a disability, although the exact conditions which qualify are not stipulated. Clearly, people who are acutely ill with schizophrenia or manic depressive disorder should not drive. Fortunately, they do not usually attempt it. Problems are more likely if your relative is recovering, and you may not be sure if it is a good idea for them to drive, particularly if they are taking medication. Most psychiatric medication interferes to some extent with the ability to drive. There are now clear guidelines on the right to drive for people with schizophrenia or manic depressive illness. Following an acute episode of schizophrenia requiring hospital admission, people must not drive a car or motorbike for six months, and their licence will only be restored when they have been free from acute symptoms during this period and if they are fully compliant with any medication prescribed. Licences are only given for 1, 2 or 3 years, and are subject to medical review on renewal. Similar rules apply to people with manic depressive disorder, and if they have frequent attacks the period in which they cannot drive may be increased to twelve months. These disorders virtually exclude sufferers from driving heavy goods vehicles, as might be imagined. Interestingly, the Driver and Vehicle Licencing Agency do not see the medication given to people for these conditions as excluding them from driving. It may be useful to talk to your relative's doctor about the problem. In extreme cases, if you cannot persuade your relative not to drive, you yourself may have to contact the DVLA. The doctor may have to do this anyway if he or she feels that public duty overrides the duty of professional confidentiality.

WHERE CAN I GET FURTHER ADVICE?

RETHINK can be a great source of support. Mind are very good at meeting requests for information, and have a range of booklets about particular topics. The responsibility for written information about rights under the Mental Health Act rests with the Hospital Managers, via their authorised agents in the hospital. Thus the hospital will have leaflets about these matters. A list of other organizations you may find useful can be found in the appendix.

Appendix

When we first wrote this book, one of the complaints of people caring for someone with severe mental illness was the almost complete lack of accessible information. We therefore included a list of useful addresses as an appendix. However, times have indeed changed, such that, if anything, there is now rather too much information. Everyone these days can have access to the internet, whether through their own connections at home, or by way of libraries or internet cafes (where staff usually enjoy helping people new to accessing it). Thus we have opted for a select list of websites that should get you started in any quest for further information.

The Association for Post Natal Illness: www.apni.org
The Association for Post Natal illness is a charity providing support for mothers suffering from postnatal psychiatric disorders.

BBC online mental health section:
www.bbc.co.uk/health/conditions/mental_health

BBC online have a health section that includes mental health pages. These carry a considerable amount of information, although its coverage is patchy..

Benefits and Work: www.benefitsandwork.co.uk/
The Benefits and Work website provides free guides about all aspects of available benefits, including disability living allowance, attendance allowance, and incapacity benefit. The website is for people with long-term physical or mental health conditions, but also for carers.

British National Formulary: www.bnf.org.uk/bnf/
The British National Formulary is now available online. This gives an extremely up to date and comprehensive account of medication available in Britain. Although the information is necessarily technical, it is clearly written, concise and accessible. To see the actual text of the formulary, you require to register.

British Association for Behavioural and Cognitive Psychotherapists:
www.babcp.org.uk
The Association is the organization responsible for accrediting
therapists who practise CBT. It publishes a directory of accredited
cognitive behavioural psychotherapists, which the public can access for
a small fee.

The British Psychological Society publishes the latest psychological
research on the causes, experiences and treatment of psychosis
www.understandingpsychosis.com

Carers UK: www.carersuk.org/Home
This is an organisation specifically for carers. Again it carries a
comprehensive range of information on the website. It covers all
aspects of caring, not just in relation to mental health.

The Citizens' Advice Bureau (www.citizensadvice.org.uk) also has a
separate advice website
www.citizensadvice.org.uk

The Court of Protection (see page 62) falls under the responsibility of
the Public Guardianship Office:
www.publictrust.gov.uk

Hyphen-21 is a small charity that promotes a number of initiatives
exemplifying basic principles of care. Its website is linked with that of
the Sainsbury Centre, which focuses particularly on Hyphen-21's
section on user involvement
www.hyphen-21.org

Institute of Mental Health Act Practitioners (IMHAP):
www.markwalton.net/
This website offers exhaustive information on legal rights under the
Mental Health Act. It provides a guide to the Mental Health Act and the
whole act is available online. One of its sections is devoted to carers,
and includes links to many useful guidelines and reports. For the
enthusiastic, the website also gives access to the evidence being
assessed by the House of Commons/House of Lords Joint Committee
on the draft mental health bill.

The Institute of Psychiatry publishes the latest research on mental
illness, together with carers' accounts
www.mentalhealthcare.org.uk

King's Fund: www.kingsfund.org.uk
The King's fund is an independent healthcare charity with the remit of
working for better health in London. It gives grants to individuals and

organisations to carry out research and development work in order to improve health policies and services.

Maca (formerly the Mental Aftercare Association) is a provider organisation. It works in partnership with other organisations, such as primary care trusts and local authorities, to run a wide range of mental health services, including community support services, advocacy services, day support services, employment training services, respite schemes for carers, forensic services for people in the criminal-justice system, supported housing and care-homes. At a hundred and twenty-five years old, it is the country's oldest community mental health charity. It also works to influence national mental health policy and improve practice in mental health care. Its website is well designed: www.maca.org.uk

Manic Depression Fellowship: www.mdf.org.uk/
The Manic Depression Fellowship is devoted to people affected by bipolar disorder, whether sufferers or carers. Once more it sees itself as being an important information resource for the public. Bipolar disorder has been something of a Cinderella within the mental health arena, reflected in the rather small amount of research, and this organisation seeks to provide as much information as possible about the condition.

Mental Health Association for Ireland: www.mentalhealthireland.ie
The Mental Health Association for Ireland is the national voluntary organisation for mental health, and works throughout Ireland. It has nearly 100 local branches.

Mental Health Care: www.mentalhealthcare.org.uk
This website is run jointly by the Institute of Psychiatry and RETHINK. It includes the latest research from the Institute of Psychiatry, together with carers' comments and their own stories.

The Mental Health Foundation: www.mentalhealth.org.uk
The Mental Health Foundation (MHF) is a long established organisation with a superb website, claimed to be the largest mental health website in the UK. The Mental Health Foundation is again devoted to lobbying for the interests of people with mental health problems. It also takes the lead in developing pilot projects. The website includes an A-Z of problems. Many of these are attached to the MHF's own fact sheets.

The Meriden Family Programme has a website that aims to be a resource for service users, families, carers and staff working in mental health services: www.Meridenfamilyprogramme.com

Mind: www.mind.org.uk
Mind is a lobbying organisation devoted to advancing the cause of people with mental health problems. It works to influence policy by campaigning and through education. It is particularly concerned with the quality of mental health services, and campaigns for them to reflect the diverse needs of people with mental health problems. The organisation has a superb website from which you can download fact sheets and booklets on a whole host of topics to do with mental illness. In addition to medical information they also provide legal guidance. In addition to the central organisation there are over 200 local Mind associations in England and Wales, so there should be one near you. The web site includes a section on news, policy and campaigns. It also provides links into a whole range of other organisations.

National electronic Library for Mental Health: www.nelmh.org/
The National electronic Library for Mental Health is a specialist library website managed by the Centre for Evidence Based Mental Health within the National electronic Library for Health. Its aim is to provide the best available evidence to answer mental health questions. The website is very well organized, and provides information on a wide range of mental health issues. There is a section on mood disorders, and the one on schizophrenic disorders includes links to the NICE schizophrenia guidelines. There is a section on evidence based treatments, which at the moment includes only antidepressants, although it will be added to later. However, it gives a detailed account of each drug.

The National Institute for Mental Health for England (NIMHE). The main sponsor of NIMHE is the Department of Health. It is responsible for supporting the implementation of positive change in mental health and mental health services. It is part of the Care Services Improvement Partnership (CSIP). It has eight development centres, through which the majority of its work is delivered. It includes a Mental Health Research Network. The NIMHE website is good on material and easier to use than the Sainsbury site.
www.nimhe.org.uk

The National Voices Forum: www.voicesforum.org.uk
The National Voices Forum describes itself as a UK user led organisation run by mad people for mad people. It includes personal web pages from people with psychotic disorders and also pages devoted to creative work and personal accounts by people who use the website. There is also a magazine called Perceptions which is becoming increasingly popular.

NHS Direct: www.nhsdirect.nhs.uk
NHS Direct is a 24 hour nurse-led telephone advice and information service and is part of the National Health Service (0845 4647). There is also an online service. This gives access among other things to a health encyclopaedia.

NSPCCInform: www.nspcc.org.uk/inform
This National Society for the Prevention of Cruelty to Children website includes a briefing paper on the welfare of children of mentally ill parents. This summarises key research and the resources available to provide support to such children.

The North Staffordshire user group is one of the larger and more successful ones around.
www.nsug.co.uk

Psychminded: Adam James, a journalist who edits the 'OpenMind' news section also runs an independent website, which carries topics and discussion items about mental health issues: www.psychminded.co.uk

The Royal College of Psychiatrists: www.rcpsych.ac.uk/
The Royal College of Psychiatrists is the professional body for psychiatrists in Britain. It is responsible for organising the profession, and before psychiatrists can become consultants they must be members of the Royal College, a status obtained by taking the Membership examination. The College has a considerable amount of mental health information on its website, including newly updated leaflets on schizophrenia and depression.

Sainsbury Centre: www.scmh.org.uk
The Sainsbury Centre is an independent charity which lobbies for improvements in mental health policy and practice. It is concerned with encouraging the development of first-rate mental health services and contributes through a programme of research and training.

Samaritans: www.samaritans.org.uk
The Samaritans is a registered charity that operates both in the UK and the Republic of Ireland. It lobbies to increase public awareness on issues concerning suicide and depression. However, its highest profile activity is a helpline for people who are suicidal or despairing (UK: 08457 90 90 90; RoI: 185060 90 90).

SANE: www.sane.org.uk
SANE was established 20 years ago following the huge public response to articles in The Times about schizophrenia by Marjorie Wallace who is now SANE's chief executive. SANE has now broadened its focus

from schizophrenia to all mental illnesses. It provides information on emotional support to people with mental health problems, their families and their carers. This is partly provided through SANELINE (0845 767 8000, which is available between midday and 2 a.m.

Scottish Association for Mental Health: www.samh.org.uk/

Scottish Development Centre for Mental Health: www.sdcmh.org.uk
The Scottish Development Centre for Mental Health aims to improve mental health and well-being for both individuals and communities in Scotland, and to improve services and supports for people with mental health problems. The centre provides services including training, information sharing and learning, research and evaluation,. It is an independent charity.

Thanks to Rogan Wolf for help with this list.

Index

Handwritten annotation at top of page: 1, 2, 3, 4, 5, 6, 7, ⑧, 9, 10, 11 12, 13, 14, 15, 16, 17, 22